THE FINEST TRADITIONS OF MY CALLING

UM, M.D.

ıditions

of My Calling

One Physician's Search for
the Renewal of Medicine

Yale UNIVERSITY PRESS

NEW HAVEN AND LONDON

Published with assistance from the foundation established
in memory of Amasa Stone Mather of the Class of 1907, Yale College.

Yale University Press books may be purchased in quantity
for educational, business, or promotional use. For information,
please e-mail sales.press@yale.edu (U.S. office) or
sales@yaleup.co.uk (U.K. office).

Set in Janson Oldstyle and Futura Bold types by Newgen North America.
Printed in the United States of America.

Library of Congress Control Number: 2015949625
ISBN 978-0-300-21140-5 (cloth : alk. paper)

A catalogue record for this book is available from the British Library.

This paper meets the requirements of ANSI/NISO Z39.48–1992
(Permanence of Paper).

10 9 8 7 6 5 4 3 2 1

AUTHOR'S NOTE

The book that you are reading contains true stories from my experiences as a physician. I changed the names and identifying details of some people to respect their privacy. The conversations in the book all come from my clear recollection of them and are not word-for-word transcripts. Instead, I retold them to evoke the feeling and meaning that was my experience.

To Elin

May I always act so as to preserve the finest traditions of my calling and may I long experience the joy of healing those who seek my help.

—*Hippocratic Oath*

CONTENTS

CONTENTS

PREFACE

You begin medical training by making promises. You swear oaths to your predecessors, to your patients, and to your creditors.

You are assigned to clinics and hospitals to learn from your betters. You listen to them, but when you see patients on your own you feel undone by all you cannot do. People fall ill in ways that startle you. Above all, ill people surprise you by placing their hopes on your unproven shoulders.

You persevere, you accrete experience, and around the time your first name is replaced by "Doctor," you become accustomed to bearing these hopes. It takes a decade or so, but you find your own place in a clinic or hospital. You start teaching students of your own. You find yourself asking what you are doing in these clinics and hospitals, where people meet each other as patients and physicians.

Patients, practitioners, and policy makers ask the same question and conclude that we need to reform the healthcare system to which we now belong. Patients routinely survive illnesses that would have felled them only a few decades ago, but they are disappointed by clinics and hospitals. They complain that receiving healthcare is too alienating and too costly. Practitioners receive salaries and social status in excess of other members of caring professions, but report high levels of fatigue and frustration. They grouse that practicing medicine has become intolerable, and discourage students from becoming physicians. Policy makers appreciate the advances of medicine, but characterize the delivery of medical services as inefficient and ineffective. They are dispirited by the inequitable distribution of care. For all these reasons, we have decided it is time to reform healthcare.

When you hear about healthcare reform, it is often described like a boat race, with a discrete beginning and a certain end. Healthcare reform is something we can achieve or complete, something we can finish. When we reach the reform finish line, practitioners will provide care that will prevent many common illnesses. If people do fall ill, efficient practitioners will provide effective care at an affordable price.

When you practice medicine, healthcare reform seems less like a well-organized race and more like being at sea on an unmarked course of indeterminate distance. You cannot recall where the starting line is and cannot envision the finish line. You feel like a crewmember on a vast ship steered by multiple captains who cannot agree on the course. As you execute the shifting priorities of the captains, you become so concerned about keeping your place on the ship that you have little time to figure out where the ship is headed.

When you are lost, it helps to retrace your journey.

• • •

In *The Finest Traditions of My Calling*, I return to the oaths I swore at the beginning of my training, and to the best traditions of medicine to which they appeal. I discuss the ways medicine advanced by embracing science, statistics, industrial engineering, customer service, and social justice and the ways medicine is being transformed by healthcare reform. The book is not intended to be comprehensive—a conspectus or summary of all the reform efforts going on in healthcare—rather, it is a narrative search for a true reform, for the renewal of medicine. The search took me from a sprawling hospital to an ancient poorhouse, an army outpost, and a medical marijuana dispensary. It is a particular account by a specific physician, reflecting upon the oaths he swore, and wondering where this ship is headed.

At present, my own place on the ship is as the director of adult inpatient psychiatry at Denver Health, an academic safety-net hospital. At times, I have been a patient, a volunteer, a student, a trainee, an ethicist, a teacher, a quality-improvement officer, a researcher, an electronic medical record builder, and an administrator. Those experiences inform this book, which is about practicing medicine during healthcare reform and searching for a finish line, a fitting port. Even, perhaps, a port where healthcare is not simply reformed, but the practice of medicine is renewed.

ACKNOWLEDGMENTS

Some kids go premed in preschool. Once they start playing doctor, they never break character. In kindergarten, they dress as physicians for Halloween. In second grade, they plate bacteria for the science fair. In fourth grade, they understand worm dissection as a practice session for gross anatomy. Not me. I finished college before I ever thought of becoming a physician.

My own preschool games occurred in my grandfather's tire store. My sisters and I would clamber up a stack of belted radials, then leap into a pile of retreads, acting out the stories of our heroes and villains. Our games always returned to the one object in the shop that did not bear the logo of a tire manufacturer, a statue of a man rendered in rebar. He stood watch in the middle of the shop. His head was thrown back, his toothless mouth loosing a scream, his hands gripping his ribs as though he were prying open an escape hatch. From beneath his ribs, rusted cogs and wheels spilled out. We knew he was a sculpture, but we were afraid to touch him. His pain created a silence that separated him from us, a separation that I wondered how to resolve.

My journey from those wordless encounters with a body in pain to working as a physician was circuitous. I would never have arrived without assistance.

My four siblings, some of whom played with me in the tire shop, are my betters. Elisabeth is a better caregiver, Mary Margaret a better writer, Anna Cate a better thinker, and Andrew a better brother. I am grateful for their company and for their spouses and children who better our family.

Among my friends, I especially thank Andy Barton, who saved my life, and Tom Buller, who taught me what it means to go on after you lose a life.

My every step was guided by teachers, including Eva Aagaard, Neil Allman, Nadia Bolz-Weber, Andrew Ciferni, Karon Dawkins, Georgette Dent, Sue Estroff, Gary Gala, Stanley Hauerwas, Tess Jones, Nancy M. P. King, Michelle Kinney, Brett McCarty, David Moore, Jennifer Nelson, Laura and Roy Nichols, Lossie Ortiz, Don Spencer, Scott Stroup, and Joel Yager.

I have the opportunity to write this only because two other teachers, Farr Curlin and Daniel Sulmasy, offered me a University of Chicago Program on Medicine and Religion Faculty Scholars Award. Funded by the Templeton Foundation, the program introduced me to my remarkable fellow scholars Michael Balboni, Amy Debaets, Lydia Dugdale, John Hardt, Aasim Padela, and Elena Salmoirago-Blotcher. Finally, the program rekindled my friendship with Warren Kinghorn, who is a model of the good physician.

I work on becoming a good physician at my clinical home, Denver Health. Denver Health is a place where one can still practice medicine—we can see a patient irrespective of his or her ability to pay while teaching students and residents—and can learn from dedicated physicians like Vince Collins, Phil Fung (who reminded me about the case of Libby Zion), Gareen Hamalian, Rebecca Hanratty, Craig Holland, Jeff Johnson, Abby Lozano, Tom MacKenzie, Melanie Rylander, Allison Sabel, Jeffrey Sankoff, and Christian Thurstone. Robert House, the director of behavioral health at Denver Health, and Robert Freedman, my department chairman at the University of Colorado, have provided sustaining encouragement and transformative opportunities since I joined the faculty.

My local editor, Bridget Rector, improved every line of this book. My literary agent, Don Fehr, answered my query letter, gave my proposal a fitting shape, and found a home for this book at Yale University Press. At Yale, Senior Executive Editor Jean Thomson Black, manuscript editor Susan Laity, and the anonymous reviewers enriched the book with their careful attention.

My parents are attentive readers who piled every table and nightstand in our home with magazines and books. Our proudest possession was a shield-shaped plaque that named us the "Library Family of the Year" for checking out more books from the public library than any other family in town. It hung on the wall of our dining room.

That plaque hangs now on the wall of my own dining room. Though our own children are compulsive readers, I suspect the only thing Eamon, Mary Clare, and Helena Frances will appreciate about this book is its completion. As involuntary passengers on our family's journey through the peculiar world of medicine, they have been subjected to call nights, post-call days, and too many dinner conversations about illness. I hope they remember us with mercy.

• • •

I distrust romances, but I could have told the story of the past fifteen years as a love story. I met my wife on the first day of orientation to medical school. I was sure we knew each other; she insisted we were strangers. I asked to sit next to her in lectures; she allowed it. We started eating lunch together on a narrow balcony overlooking the morgue. As we ate, we talked. She excelled at medical school; I struggled. She knew she wanted to be a physician; I thought of dropping out.

I would have left med school if I had not feared that it would mean never seeing Elin again. I desired to see her every day, but doubted desire. One night, when I should I have been reading biochemistry, I read Norman MacLean's *Young Men and Fire*, his account of Montana smokejumpers. Like medical students, the smokejumpers were idealistic and young. MacLean observed that for most of the smokejumpers, there were girls they met at bars and drank with and girls at home that they married. He described a girl at home this way: "She was strong like him, and a great walker like him, and she could pack forty pounds all day. He thought of her as walking with him now and shyly showing her love by offering to pack one of his double-tools. He was thinking he was returning her love by shyly refusing to let her." Reading that passage, I knew Elin was the girl you take on the long walk, the girl with whom you shyly share your burdens, and the woman you marry. We married as third year med students, and she gave birth to our first child when we were fourth year med students. It was a daring time to set out together, but twelve years and three children later, we are still walking together, and this book grew from the life we share.

THE FINEST TRADITIONS OF MY CALLING

As you become a physician, you feel as if you are learning to see people as a compendium of parts and a source of income: parts and money.

No one pulls you aside during training and tells you this plainly.

Just the same, you learn, as I did in the first month of medical school when my very first patient died before I could ask her her name.

Before meeting her, I had not had personal contact with any real patients, just abstractions of patients. The first weeks of medical school were filled with a series of PowerPoint presentations. We watched as animated arrows flashed and the Krebs cycle generated energy, or molecules bound to receptors and cell membranes opened, like the locks of a canal, so that potassium and sodium ions could travel in and out of a cell. Professors discussed the body as a series of simple machines. As they spoke, we dozed in the darkened lecture hall. When the fluorescent lights flickered on, we rubbed our eyes, collected our backpacks, and stumbled upstairs to the anatomy lab, where we dissected the upper back of a corpse while avoiding its dead eyes.

After a few weeks of this, the medical school sent us away for week-long apprenticeships in the practices of rural primary care physicians. We were going to see real patients! On the first Monday, I woke up early and put on my least-wrinkled shirt and an almost-matching tie. I covered these up with a short white poly-cotton-blend lab coat. In the mirror, I looked more like a busboy than a physician. To shore up my authority and clarify my role, I filled my pockets with medical tools—a penlight, reflex hammer, stethoscope, and tuning fork— that I did not know how to wield.

I arrived before the first patient, and the physician greeted me in his consultation room. He was young, but his office was old-fashioned, the walls dotted with diplomas and framed Norman Rockwell lithographs. His oversized wooden desk faced two leather chairs. As I sat before him, he said he liked having students. "It gives the patient someone to talk to while I am seeing the previous patient. You can sit and listen, while I keep moving. I have to move, move, move if I want the lights to stay on." So we began, and I followed his rhythm. I would go in first, fumbling through the patient's history and exam for a few minutes. Then the physician would enter while knocking, striding from the door to the patient's back and placing his stethoscope under the shirt without invitation. "Take a deep breath. Good. And again." While he lifted his stethoscope off the chest, he would advise more meds, or a new med, as he marked a billing code on the patient's chart. With these codes he monetized every minute of his day. He later told me that if he spent ten minutes with a return patient, he generated a profit. If he spent twelve minutes, he broke even. If he spent fourteen minutes, he lost money. His profits depended on efficiently moving patients through the clinic.

That afternoon, in the midst of this bustle, the office phone rang. The adjacent hospital was calling. "A patient of your practice is coming to the hospital by ambulance. Can the physician come?" The physician had a double-booked morning, so he sent me instead. "It will be good for you to see how the Emergency Room works," he said, and patted me out the door.

I was eager to see an acutely ill patient instead of the people with chronic diseases who filled his exam rooms. I ran across the parking lot, my tools dully rattling in my pockets. When I arrived, the Emergency Department was tensely quiet as the nurses prepared for the arrival of the patient. Then the paramedics arrived, pushing an aluminum gurney with an unconscious woman cradled between its rails. The lead paramedic announced his cargo: "Fifty-six-year-old woman. History of hypertension and diabetes. Collapsed at work twelve minutes ago. BP 50 over nothing. Pulse 52. ST elevations in V1–6." As they spoke, they wheeled the unconscious woman toward ED-1, the largest bay in the Emergency Department, the bay where the tools to revive the most critically ill patients were arrayed.

The woman's dress was cleaved open by sterilized scissors to bare her chest. A pair of physicians and a trio of nurses descended on her. Together they moved about her, announcing their actions to one another: "Cardiac monitor in place. IV access obtained. Labs drawn. Administer streptokinase." Using their skills in concert, they localized the failing part: her heart.

The diagnosis was apparent to everyone in the room but the patient and me. She was unconscious, and I was ignorant. I stood still, afraid that my movements would be disruptive, while the paramedics, nurses, and physicians worked. They spoke to one another in code: "STEMI. Unresponsive. Won't make it for transfer to perc." They worked together through a familiar algorithm, following a lifesaving script. Despite their coordination, the patient's heart never regained its rhythm.

As the exhausted physicians and nurses left the room, they finally departed from the script. "Tombstoned. You ever seen that before?" one of them asked. "Broken pump. Too bad," the other commented. The woman's parts had failed her.

Nursing assistants moved in. They cleaned the woman's body, removing the medical waste that littered her exposed thorax. I stood at the foot of the bed, uncertain what to do. I averted my eyes and noticed a stain on my new white coat.

As I looked for something with which to clean it, a nurse approached me and said, "Her son is in the waiting room, but the physicians are busy with another patient who just came in. Can you talk with the son and tell him what happened?"

Too afraid to say no, I mumbled, "Sure," and then made a quick call to the physician's office, seeking guidance about how to tell a son his mother was dead. The physician's receptionist put me through to the clinic nurse. "The physician is busy seeing patients, so you will have to do it yourself," she instructed. "It's what physicians do."

I wanted to do what physicians do. I entered the Family Waiting Room and asked for the "son of our emergency patient." A young African American man about my age was standing in the middle of the room, rocking from side to side. He had been called from his work as a cook and was still wearing his own white coat. Through tears, he asked, "Where is my mother? What happened to her? Where is the doctor?" I stammered, realizing I did not even know his mother's name. All I could do was repeat what I had heard. "Her heart failed her," I said. "Her heart failed her. She died." He let out a cry, and only then did I learn my patient's name.

"She's not a 'her'! She's my mama. Her name is Gloria. Gloria! What will I do without her?"

• • •

That morning I had watched paramedics, nurses, and physicians working efficiently, if unsuccessfully, to save Gloria's life.

I had also seen how they looked at Gloria. In the Emergency Room, they saw a massive heart attack and worked efficiently to treat the broken part. As they did so, her primary care physician was in his office, where patients were viewed as billing codes. He knew that if he left his outpatient practice to see Gloria, he would lose the revenue from his scheduled appointments. If he visited her in the hospital, he could not bill for providing services to Gloria or her family because, by the rules of Gloria's insurance, only the hospital could bill for a physician's services. So the physician stayed in the clinic to keep the lights on. As he labored, Gloria's son lost his mother.

Parts and money—too often that is what we physicians see when we look at patients. What is broken? Can it be patched or does it need to be replaced? How much can I bill for the procedure? How much of that fee will I take home?

The questions Gloria's son asked that morning were very different. He wanted to know where his mother was, what had happened to her, where the physician was, and what he would do without her. He also wanted to know why I did not know her name. I tried to respond as best I could, but my words did not satisfy him or me. Instead, our meeting was another alienating encounter in a society divided by class and race. I was so confused by it that I began asking myself what we hope for when we call in the doctor.

Everyone has a story about medicine's failures. When you need medical assistance, it is difficult to find any physician, let alone the right physician. The queues are long, the costs high, the outcomes inconsistent, and the experiences alienating. Everyone also seems to have a solution—prioritize primary care, promote evidence-based medicine, provide universal insurance, pay for performance, push down costs.

As I continued my training, I sought out the most promising initiatives to "fix" medicine, its finest traditions, and tried most of them out. Along the way, I learned that few of them address the questions of Gloria's son, for almost all fail to take into account the lessons of history, of how medicine moved toward the system we have today.

The advances in knowledge in twentieth-century medicine began with a change in physicians' self-perception in the nineteenth century; modern medicine was born when physicians learned to see like scientists. And I suspect that medicine will advance once more only when physicians change their self-perception again.[1] In contemporary medicine, the underlying problem is that we see the wrong things or, rather, not all of the right things when we look at patients. My encounters with Gloria and her son led me to seek better ways of seeing patients and of being seen by patients. I am trying to find a renewed vision for medicine.

Medical training is a series of vision lessons. In each encounter with a patient, you learn something about being with the ill. On my first day in that rural clinic, I learned that a physician does not need to know the name of his patient and that an unskilled student might have to tell a son that his mother was dead. In the medical community, knowing names and communicating with families were less important than generating money by trying to fix faltering parts.

I also learned that even when physicians and nurses and paramedics work together as a team, even when they follow an evidence-based script in pursuit of consistent outcomes, the care they offer is often dehumanizing.

Fifteen years later, I still remember the name of the rural physician, even though we spent only a few weeks together, but I cannot remember Gloria's real name; I remember only that her son knew it and I did not. I can remember the name of a physician but not of the first person I watched die. I worry about what that says about me. Am I broken, or is medicine?

I suspect that the answers are yes and yes.

• • •

To write this book, I had to give Gloria a name and re-create dialogue from memory, which means that the story of Gloria is a representation of an event rather than a transcription. However, the details of her death came from records I made at the time. During my training, I wrote letters, sporadically kept a journal, and composed case presentations. I drew upon those occasional writings for this book. As with Gloria and her son, I do not remember the names of all the people I write about. Even when I do remember the names of the people I write about, I changed their names and identifying details to preserve their privacy. I hesitated to alter the names and details, but I did so for two reasons. First, these stories belong not to me but to the people I have been privileged to meet. Ideally, I might contact each person and seek his or her permission, but these episodes occurred over two decades, and it would be impossible for me to find all the patients. Many are deceased. Second, these stories concern only a portion of each person's story, his or her time as a patient with me, so I tell them as I experienced them while remembering that they are vignettes, not the entire story of any particular person. I tell these stories from my perspective, flawed as that may be. Any resulting errors or mistakes belong on my ledger, not on those of the people I describe.

The dialogue reflects my memory of the feeling and meaning of conversations as I experienced them, aided in some instances by personal reflections, letters, or journals I kept at the time.

The physicians and teachers I do name have consented to my doing so; I thank them for their generosity.

Many of these stories date from when I was in medical school and residency, but some happened when I began practicing as a psychiatrist. As I tell my friends in other specialties, most of medicine is beginning to resemble psychiatry because it is less concerned with trying to save people like Gloria from dying of a heart attack in the Emergency Department and more with attending to her chronic heart disease back in the office. There are no cures for chronic diseases like diabetes and hypertension, so the measures of a physician's success are changing. At our best, psychiatrists are ahead of that change. The majority of our patients have chronic diseases whose cures are in the future; our present success is best measured by our ability to persuade people to seek health rather than by telling them the right thing to do or by performing a procedure upon them.

• • •

I interact with colleagues in other specialties every day because I spend my days entrenched in a contemporary hospital. On the floor below our ward, surgeons are bravely using the latest instruments in operating rooms. On the floor above our ward, internists are maintaining the faltering bodies of ill people through techniques only dreamed of a half-century ago. I travel often between our ward and these other particular, peculiar spaces of contemporary medicine as a physician consultant, teacher, and administrator.

As I move between these wards, I am struck by the confusion within medicine. The units shine, the surgical instruments are precise, the medical techniques are novel, and yet the physicians are discouraged. Physician burnout, early retirement, and suicide are increasing.[2] Most physicians report that they would discourage a student from joining the profession. No one thinks the current state is acceptable, so reforms are forever being proposed, studied, implemented, and abandoned. Few of these reforms address the problem I consider fundamental: that we no longer see our patients as people. In fact, most reforms shift the frame ever farther away from the individual patient to the health of populations by attempting to standardize outcomes on a population basis. We are encouraged to count something, rather than to see someone.

Many reforms also shift the authority of healthcare decisions away from physicians. So why do I write about physicians? After all, more than ever before, healthcare requires the kind of coordinated teamwork I saw in the attempts to save Gloria. Nurses deliver most of the care in hospitals. If you want to select a good hospital, you should choose it based on the ability and stability of the nursing staff, rather than on the achievements of its physicians. Occupational and physical therapists rehabilitate most serious injuries. If you want a torn ligament repaired, make sure you have a good physical therapist as well as a good orthopedic surgeon. Social workers transform the trajectory of a child in foster care; if you want to improve the health of small children, social workers can matter more than pediatricians. Pharmacists prevent life-threatening medication errors: if you are going to take a dangerous medication like warfarin, find a skilled pharmacist as well as a highly trained internist.

As each of these professions develops its own specialized approaches and knowledge bases, practitioners are often required to obtain a doctorate in the field. We can no longer speak about "doctors" in healthcare and be sure of what we mean. In my job, I work with chaplains, nurses, nurse practitioners, pharmacists, physical therapists, psychologists, and others who hold doctorates. All of them can be rightly addressed as "Doctor." Members of each of these professions can improve the health and well-being of an ill person, often more effectively than a physician.

I write about physicians in part because I am a physician and in part because, at least for now, physicians still make the important decisions about what goes on in medical care. Physicians admit patients to hospitals where nurses care for them, assign patients to the rehab where physical therapists help them regain mobility, refer children to social workers who intervene in their lives, and order the medications a pharmacist compounds and monitors. Among practitioners, physicians are disproportionately represented in the leadership of hospitals, universities, insurers, and regulators. In the coming years, physicians may play a smaller role in the healthcare system, but for now the habits of physicians remain a critical factor in healthcare reform. To transform healthcare, we must engage physicians.

Every physician is a particular, unique individual. There is, as the saying goes, no vision from nowhere. I was a reader before I was a physician, and so my own vision is shaped by a love of history, literature, philosophy, and theology. These books guided my vision and taught me the meaning of events like Gloria's death. I share my search in the hope that if we physicians can learn how to attend to patients as fellow creatures, we can renew the practice of medicine.

"Doc, you remember our handshake? The Nussbaum handshake? First you slap, then you shake, then you slide! It's the Nussbaum sandshake, the Nussnutt landrake, the Fussbutt bandlake, the Cussbutt taketake!"

Martha is on the unit again, slinging speech, her words clanging off each other in a rhythm only she can follow. She spent decades as a nurse at a hospital across town, but these days she is mostly a patient, either on our unit or in the apartment she shares with her sister.

Once a year she becomes manic. Her mania starts with a walking rhythm. She calls up old boyfriends. Starts writing poetry about the old boyfriends. Then the rhythm accelerates and she stops sleeping. Soon she barricades the door to her bedroom. Her sister pleads with her to come out, sliding tablets of lithium underneath the door, but Martha crushes them under her dancing heels. Her sister calls a case manager or a police officer to coax Martha out of her room. Together they deliver Martha to the hospital, and we bring her back into a rhythm the rest of us can follow.

Twice a year she becomes depressed. This rhythm starts out slow and, unbidden, becomes halting. She falls into stop-time. She calls up no one. She rarely leaves her apartment. She writes nothing. She sleeps around the clock. She leaves the door to her room open but lies on her bed, thick tears salting the nicotine-carved crevices of her face, and eats nothing. Her sister brings her, slump-shouldered, to the hospital, and we try to interest her in life again.

I have been Martha's physician for all her hospitalizations over the past several years. She is one of our regulars, so, in a way, I know her better than any of her other physicians do. Her outpatient physicians see her quarterly for fifteen-minute visits in which they focus on symptoms and medication effects, but when Martha is on the unit,

I see her at least once and often twice a day. Some of the regulars resent being hospitalized and greet me tersely. Others, like Martha, grace me with their affection.

A few hospitalizations back, Martha formalized her affection for me with a handshake. I shake hands with all my patients, but it is usually a simple affair: a firm grip, eye contact, a modest pump, and a surreptitious squirt of hand sanitizer afterward. Most of my handshakes communicate little more than a greeting and a fear of contagion. Martha managed to communicate that I knew her and that she knew me. She called our handshake the "Nussbaum handshake," or the "dream shake." Whenever we met, whether she was manic or depressed, she offered me her hand, and I followed her lead. Shake. Slide and shake. Pinky swears. Fist-bump. Explosion. By the end of the handshake, I would know how she was doing. When manic, Martha filigreed the dream shake with hip-shimmies and then repeated it again and again. When depressed, Martha limped through the dream shake: a simple shake and slide could drag on for a minute without ever crescendoing into a fist-bump and explosion. The rest of our interaction simply refined the initial communication Martha made through the dream shake.

One day I was sitting with Martha, and she gave me a drawing. On a piece of construction paper she had written, "The Nussbaum Dream Shake," across the top. Below the title were numbered instructions for our handshake: 1. Shake. 2. Slide and shake. 3. Pinky swear. 4. Fist bump. 5. EXPLOSION!!! As she talked about the shake, I wondered about its dream component; how did Martha dream about me? In her dreams, was I a jailer, a friend, a lover?

I knew I could be none of those things to Martha, but then what roles were left? What does it mean to know someone as her physician, to receive her secret handshake? As I pondered these questions, my eye caught the clock. An important personage was downstairs, and I was late for his scheduled talk. I apologized to Martha, promised to return, and rode the elevator down to one of the hospital classrooms.

The basement conference room looked like any other. Rows of stacking chairs faced a raised podium behind which a man wearing a blue blazer stood like a prep school chapel speaker, except that instead of having an altar behind him, he had a screen on which to project his PowerPoint presentation. At the back of the room was an urn with coffee. I collected a burnt cup of coffee and a stale cookie. Lunch. I found a seat and tuned in to the speaker.

His slides were different from those of last month's speaker, but they followed the same rhetorical script. Healthcare must be transformed. Old ways are dying. Disruptive innovations are afoot. Creative destruction is occurring. Revolution is at hand. The speakers always have a theory about how to fix medicine. That day the theory was efficiency itself. Efficiency in what? He never really said. Efficiency for its own sake, then. The speaker was an efficiency expert. He had studied the efficient delivery models of other industries. He told us that we have no patients, only customers. He said that we were not physicians but providers of healthcare services. He explained that we were a part of the healthcare industry, the largest industry in the country, not the medical profession, and we must adopt the efficient practices of other industries.

We get this kind of talk a lot. I never understand why the speakers are so certain, yet working so hard to convince us. If the revolution has arrived, why are you trying to convince us? Revolutions require no consent from the overthrown.

In fact, ever since I entered medical school at the University of North Carolina, I have been listening to these kinds of talks. At first, I found them exhilarating. When I enrolled at Chapel Hill, the talks were about how the human genome project would transform medicine. We were told that by the beginning of residency, we would be sequencing the genome of each patient. Residency began, and we were quietly told that sequencing had little clinical utility because knowing the base pairs of a person's DNA is a bit like translating every third page of an instruction manual; the knowledge cannot be used to build something.

Halfway through medical school, the speakers starting talking about how stem cells would allow us to regrow injured organs in petri dishes. We were told that by the end of residency, we could grow new pancreases for diabetics. Residency ended, and we were told that while the cells could be grown in petri dishes, they were too unstable for humans.

At least the hopes shared in medical school were scientific. The speakers were physicians or scientists who believed that a line of research they were pursuing would soon improve human health. Everyone admired the speakers' commitment to the scientific method, even if their evidence was preliminary.

Since leaving medical school, I have found that while the talks go on, the topics have changed. By the time I finished residency in 2009 and began attending basement talks at the hospital where I now work, the speakers were lecturing not on scientific breakthroughs but on changes in healthcare financing and delivery. Each was seeking consent for a purported revolution. Each offered a slogan ("In God We Trust. All others bring outcome data."). Instead of pursuing new science, they wanted us to figure out how to implement the knowledge we had. Evidence-based medicine would synthesize the results of scientific studies. Comparative-effectiveness research would determine the best treatments. Electronic medical records would improve data gathering and prevent errors. The patient-centered medical home would reduce costly hospitalizations and increase patient compliance. Patient-centered outcomes research would measure the things that really mattered to patients. This decade of excited talk about revolution, creative destruction, and transformation culminated in legislation, such as the Affordable Care Act, which financed many of these initiatives.

After years of diligent attendance at the basement talks, I grew ambivalent about their ability to effect change, and the thought of sitting through another one often gives me a preemptive stomachache. Attending the basement talks now feels like visiting a restaurant that changes its menu too often. You are lured by the novelty, but you always leave unsatisfied because a chef needs more than a trendy recipe to make a decent meal. Just as food fads hurry through restaurant kitchens, our basement speakers are often promoting the latest fad favored by medical journals and government regulators.

The speakers come around to hospitals and medical schools when the preliminary results are promising, but we never hear from them after their hopes are dashed in the follow-up trials.

So while I sat listening to the day's basement speaker wax eloquent about efficiency, that day's innovation du jour, my mind skipped from astronaut ice cream to fondue pots to molecular gastronomy. All these "innovations" have also had their moment, and, admittedly, they all had more appeal than my coffee-and-cookie lunch. Since I was determined to stick out the lecture, I looked for something to distract me from my hunger. There was not much to see in the basement. No art adorned the walls. No windows opened to the natural world. There were only bulletin boards. Most were covered with A3 and Pareto charts, but a few bore italicized quotations. One of these caught my eye. Attributed to Sir William Osler, it read, "The value of experience is not in seeing much, but in seeing wisely."

Seeing much, huh? I do that every day. Every physician I know does that every day. And we still use the metaphor of Osler's aphorism. Before I examine patients in the hospital, I tell the staff that I am "going to see my patients now." The hospital always wants me to see more patients, because the more patients I see, the more bills I submit. Physicians have accepted this increased load because the more bills we submit, the more income we bring home. So hospitals are forever asking for physicians to evaluate more patients in the clinic, to perform more procedures in the operating room, and to examine more patients in the hospital. Seeing much is what we do.

In fact, seeing much is what we have been training physicians to do for the past hundred years. Medical education has favored "seeing much" through a high volume of experiences at least since the 1910 report on medical education written by Abraham Flexner. Flexner's *Report* transformed American medicine by encouraging mastery through repeated experience. Before Flexner, most physicians trained through apprenticeships to practicing physicians in a particular community. Many medical schools were less rigorous than the high schools in their community, and Flexner's *Report* characterized all but 6 of America's 155 medical schools as inadequate.[1] The leading exception was Osler's own Johns Hopkins University School of Medicine. Although Osler himself disputed some of the characterizations of Johns Hopkins in the *Report*, he agreed with its central tenet—that the education of physicians should be rigorous and based on science. After Flexner, Hopkins and its Oslerian philosophy became the paradigm for all of medicine. Physicians now train at centralized research universities and teaching hospitals, where they work as part of shifting teams of physicians, before practicing in a particular community.

In the system spawned by Flexner, physicians leave whatever particular communities they may belong to so they can spend a decade or more developing specialized skills. Undergraduates are advised to attend the best medical school that accepts them, even if it is across the country in a place where the student knows no one. Residents and fellows are advised to train at the most prestigious program they can "match at," even if it means uprooting a spouse from his or her employment. So instead of training with the general surgeon in his or her hometown, the student trains with the otolaryngologist at the nearest medical school—or, even better, with the renowned otolaryngologist at a distant research university. But once the student is there the faculty explains that otolaryngology is far too broad a field, so the student becomes a thyroid and parathyroid microvascular otolaryngologist.

As their medical training extends, physicians leave their communities behind while narrowing their vision to an ever more specific part of the body, which they control through medical procedures. The student becomes a physician who follows the thyroid and parathyroid organs. If the patient has other concerns, he or she will need to see someone else. The lasting effects of Flexner's *Report* include an explosion of medical knowledge and a series of technical advances, but also a fraying of the ties between physicians and communities. We belong to the hospitals in which we train and practice.

As physicians came, over the past century, to understand themselves as scientists, medical training changed first to focus on the volume of experiences and then to use population-based data to standardize their diagnoses and treatments. There is much good in such standardization. Who would want to return to a world where prescribed medicines had widely divergent amounts of active medications? Where each physician treated a particular condition based only on his or her personal experience? Where a patient stayed in the hospital simply for as long as the physician felt it necessary? But one can have too much of a good thing, and standardization can start to resemble monoculture, the cultivation of a single crop at the expense of life's diversity.

When the speakers come to the hospital's basement with proposals to renew medicine, they usually propose further standardizing physician performance and patient outcomes. The efficiency expert identified himself as an advocate of quality improvement, or QI. At the time, I was just learning about QI. I knew it was the most widely embraced proposal to renew medicine, endorsed by every major medical society, required by residency programs, and enacted by legislation. The speaker told us that quality improvement excels at preventing common mistakes. QI personnel develop behavioral "nudges" to promote hand washing among clinicians. They create checklists to prevent surgical complications. They turn evidence-based guidelines into order sets for physicians to follow.

All these practices have real merit, but they belong firmly to the category of seeing much. The goal is the best possible outcome for the most people, assessed by seeking signals from large datasets and developing universal findings before implementing them in particular communities. So when I discharge a patient from the hospital, I am judged on how closely my documentation meets national standards, not on whether a patient feels well or has been restored to health. As I practice, I often feel like a technician following a protocol, and I start to see patients in terms of outcome measures, another version of seeing much. In these arrangements, my authority as a physician derives from seeing much, from being able to employ a specialized knowledge.

I suppose this made sense when knowledge was difficult to come by, but specialized knowledge is now easily obtained. Computers excel at building knowledge databases beyond human capacity. If being a physician is simply a question of knowing much, then physicians will become increasingly unnecessary as databases grow in their scope and interpretative power. An entry-level smartphone can access more knowledge than any physician. To the extent that medicine is about specialized knowledge derived from large population samples, it can be turned into evidence-based medicine and decision-tree algorithms, and the physicians who practice such medicine can ultimately be replaced by databases. When those databases are eventually united with technical skills, providers with more specialized knowledge and more technical ability to consistently employ that knowledge will replace physicians.

Cue up the scary robot music.

The robots do not scare me, however, because whatever robots can do well, they should do. Robots can already sort, count, and dispense medication; they may soon compound and even select the appropriate medication for some conditions. Robots can assist pathologists and radiologists through visual-recognition software today, and they may soon automatically interpret many routine images. Robots can allow physicians to remotely examine patients today and may soon perform portions of the examination themselves. If physicians are simply people with specialized knowledge, then we ought to be replaced by robots. Someone will eventually train a robot to perform thyroid and parathyroid microvascular surgery.

And then what will be left for physicians to do? It may be the other half of Osler's aphorism: See wisely.

• • •

The speaker finished talking. The lights came up, the universal sign that we were being released from our stiff seats. I walked upstairs, thinking of the speaker, of robots, of Osler, of Martha, and of food. I stopped by my office, dug a handful of almonds out of a desk drawer, and looked up Osler's words. Osler was invoked often during my training—many medical schools have Osler Societies dedicated to medical humanism, and the coffee shop at my medical school was the Osler Café—but I never really learned much about him. I knew he was a famous physician of old, but I had read his aphorisms rather than his essays. His aphorisms always seemed aspirational—speaking to the best of being a physician and suggesting the way medicine ought to be. The yearning aphorisms, like the one on the conference room wall, suggested a way out of seeing much, a way out of cranking a queue of ill patients through the healthcare factory. We could follow wisdom's call, we could see wisely, if we only followed Osler's advice.

Searching online, I found the words in a commencement speech Osler gave in 1894, sixteen years before Flexner published his report, addressed to a graduating group of army surgeons. In between suggesting possible research topics based on the posts to which they were likely to be assigned, Osler named the army surgeons' ability to move frequently as an advantage of their enlistment, saying, "Permanence of residence, good undoubtedly for the pocket, is not always best for wide mental vision in the physician." He consoled the graduates that since they would move often, they would be "seeing much in many places." He admitted that having no fixed home could isolate a physician, but if a surgeon grew weary of a remote outpost and felt it limited his learning, Osler counseled, "Comfort may be derived from a knowledge that some of the best work of the profession has come from men whose clinical field was limited but well-tilled. The important thing is to make the lesson of each case tell on your education. The value of experience is not in seeing much, but in seeing wisely. . . . In a ten or fifteen years' service, travelling with seeing eyes and hearing ears, and carefully kept note-books, just think what a store-house of clinical material may be at the command of any one of you—material not only valuable in itself to the profession, but of infinite value to you personally in its acquisition, rendering you painstaking and accurate, and giving you, year by year, an increasing experience."[2] I was surprised. In my initial reading of the aphorism, I had assumed that Osler was sharply distinguishing between seeing wisely and seeing much. Reading his essay, I realized that Osler considered seeing much to be a requirement for seeing wisely. His counsel to the army surgeons was to leave particular communities in search of experience, of seeing much.

Although most of the address is taken up with general advice, toward the end it becomes clear that Osler had a particular example in mind. Osler closed by telling the graduating army surgeons about a nineteenth-century army surgeon named William Beaumont, a physician who truly saw much. Beaumont, like Osler himself, was a dedicated observer of the physiology of the body. From medical school lectures, I vaguely recalled that Beaumont had earned a place in the history of medicine because of his groundbreaking work on the process of digestion, which stemmed from a peculiar collaboration with a young Canadian named Alexis Bidagan dit St-Martin.

On June 6, 1822, St-Martin was visiting Mackinaw Island at the northern tip of Michigan's lower peninsula. The island was home to the main trading post of John Jacob Astor's American Fur Company, and St-Martin was a nineteen-year-old *coureur de bois* in the employ of the company. Given the island's importance to the fur trade, it was protected by members of the United States Army stationed at Fort Michilimackinac. One day St-Martin was shot in the stomach, and Beaumont, the fort's resident physician, was called in to care for him. To Beaumont's surprise, St-Martin's injury had not proved fatal. Instead, his broken part had healed itself in an odd way: St-Martin's stomach formed a fistula, a communicating passage between his stomach and his abdominal wall, at the site of the wound. Beaumont tried to close the fistula but failed.[3]

As Beaumont gazed into St-Martin's open fistula, he saw an opportunity; by means of this anomaly he could study how food is digested in the stomach. Beaumont initially studied the operations of St-Martin's fistula at Fort Michilimackinac. When the army eventually decided it could no longer subsidize Beaumont's experiment and St-Martin's recovery, Beaumont moved St-Martin into his own home. There he kept St-Martin immobile and starved him for days at a time in order to conduct experiments on digestion. Once St-Martin's stomach was completely empty, Beaumont would insert foodstuffs—a partial list from Beaumont's notebook includes animal spinal marrow, apple dumplings, fresh beef suet, Irish potatoes, mellow peaches, old strong cheese, and solid hog's bone—through a glass funnel placed inside the fistula and remove the foodstuffs at varying intervals to assess how they had been altered by their time in St-Martin's stomach. Eventually, Beaumont came to an understanding of the mechanisms of digestion, earned international renown, and inaugurated a physician-patient relationship that seems like a perverse model for contemporary medicine.

Beaumont at times succored St-Martin, nursing him to health, and at other times starved him and exploited him, paying the illiterate St-Martin to participate in experiments but never sharing the book royalties and speaking fees that were generated through his work. Hampered by his physical disability and alcoholism, St-Martin struggled throughout his life to find employment other than as a research subject for Beaumont. On several occasions, St-Martin fled from Beaumont, and the physician gave chase to the patient of whom he had seen so much but wanted to see still more.

Osler praised Beaumont's efforts at the end of his speech, telling the graduating army surgeons, "William Beaumont is indeed a bright example in the annals of the Army Medical Department, and there is no name on its roll more deserving to live in the memory of the profession of this country." Osler praised the "persistence with which for eight years Beaumont pursued the subject, except during two intervals when St. Martin escaped to his relatives in Lower Canada. . . . The determination to sift the question thoroughly, to keep at it persistently until the truth was reached, is shown in every one of the 238 experiments that he has recorded. The opportunity presented itself, the observer had the necessary mental equipment and the needed store of endurance to carry to a successful termination a long and laborious research."[4] Osler praised Beaumont for his persistence and endurance—his 238 experiments—without mentioning the persistence and endurance of St-Martin. He never acknowledged why St-Martin might have fled.

Osler's fascination with Beaumont was no commencement day lark. He published a separate essay on Beaumont's experiments, and his biographers say that when Osler taught students about gastric physiology, he regaled them with tales of St-Martin, whom Osler called "old fistulous Alexis, the old sinner."[5] He routinely asked his students where St-Martin's stomach should reside when its owner, the now aged St-Martin, died. Although St-Martin outlived Beaumont, Osler took up Beaumont's cause, saying it would be a shame for St-Martin's stomach to decompose in a rural cemetery. St-Martin's stomach belonged, Osler insisted, in the United States Army Museum in Washington, D.C.

This was also not idle chatter between a teacher and his students. Osler maintained a correspondence with the local physician in the town where St-Martin lived out his last days, seeking news of St-Martin's health. Osler thought often of St-Martin's stomach and desired to perform an autopsy on the elderly subject, but St-Martin and his family concluded that they wanted no further role in medical research. When St-Martin died, on June 20, 1888, Osler received a telegram telling him that he would not be allowed to perform the autopsy. St-Martin's family refused all offers of money for his fistulous stomach, his famous part. Instead, they buried St-Martin's body below two feet of stones and six feet of dirt to ward off grave robbers and physicians, groups that were often one and the same at that time. Neighbors kept watch over the grave armed with muskets to give St-Martin the peaceful rest he never received in life.

Is that what it means to see much? To be so enamored of learning how the parts of the body work that you hound a fellow human beyond the grave? Apparently so, because every few years a medical journal will publish an article commemorating the store of knowledge generated from old fistulous Alexis.[6]

Through such articles Osler remains the most celebrated physician in recent memory, acclaimed as the father of contemporary medicine. Even though Osler never developed a novel treatment or cured an illness, his words still adorn hospital walls because of his renown as a master teacher. He gave addresses that are still read by aspiring and practicing physicians. He was the first medical educator to take students out of lecture halls and to the bedsides of ill patients. He developed the first residency program. He was a founding physician of the Johns Hopkins University School of Medicine, the first truly contemporary medical school. He perfected the contemporary medical teaching service, in which a medical student, intern, junior resident, chief resident, and fellow follow an attending physician like climbers following a leader as they ascend a ladder, each examining the team's patient and sharing responsibility for the patient's care. Osler's ladder was the model praised in Flexner's *Report* as the way to reform medicine, so, in a way, it was fitting that it was Osler's words that distracted me from the basement speaker's own talk of reform. After all, that basement room was called the Osler Classroom.

• • •

A contemporary hospital can seem like an expansive Osler Classroom. Osler remains the kind of physician the basement speakers desire to be. He is widely remembered as a tireless teacher, a perceptive physician, a heartfelt humanist. Osler is credited with achieving the grand synthesis: a medicine that is at once rigorously scientific and deeply humane. Story after story about Osler credits him with being a physician who cared for his patients and who recognized the humanity of each one; in portraits, he is often portrayed, without irony, with the attributes of a saint. Osler's hands bore prosector's warts (what dermatologists call tuberculosis verrucosa cutis)—tubercular warts from the autopsies he conducted—physical marks of suffering for his work that are analogues of a saint's stigmata.[7]

Is this what physicians are supposed to be? Scientist-saints? Martyrs for medicine? When I read about Alexis St-Martin, Beaumont and Osler did not strike me as saints or martyrs. At best, they sounded like benefactors, but the relationship could more accurately be described as that between scientist and subject. When we consider the lengths that these physicians went to access the most intimate parts of the man's body, we might even see them in a more sinister light. Social mores change, but I doubt it was ever common to post armed guards around the bodies of elderly, illiterate, disabled Canadian fur traders. In fact, historians recently learned that Osler developed a way to conduct covert autopsies when a patient or a family would not consent. By making small incisions behind the scrotum or within the vaginal vault of a deceased person, Osler could remove organs from the abdomen and thorax of deceased patients for his collection of diseased specimens, and then sew up the body for burial without anyone knowing.[8] Historians also estimate that during Osler's tenure about half the cadavers used by students at John Hopkins were obtained illegally.[9] The muskets of St-Martin's family appear to have been necessary.

In my medical specialty, psychiatry, questions of exploitation remain relevant. My patient Martha, for example, could read, but she too was elderly and disabled. She would have been easy to exploit. She lived on the margins of society. She was often confused. She was ill more often than she was well. She had no parents, spouse, or children who would mourn her. She had only her sister.

And she had me. What was the nature of our relationship? Was I her friend? Her savior? Was I the scientist studying her body the way Beaumont studied St-Martin's body? Was she in some way my subject? Who are a physician and a patient when they meet each other? These are the questions to ask.

Six months after listening to the basement speaker deliver his talk about efficiency, and still thinking about Osler's aphorism, I received a call from Martha's sister. Through tears, she said, "Martha died last week. Pneumonia. Before she passed, she wanted me to tell you good-bye." I thanked her for the call, talked a few minutes more, hung up the phone, and cried at my desk.

No more Martha. No more dream shakes.

She was no longer around for me to ask who we really are to each other when we meet as physician and patient.

But she left me with memories and a question: What would it mean for a physician to see a person wisely? I had looked up Osler's words because I thought they pointed the way to a practice of medicine that was both humanistic and scientific, a way to explain a day that included caring for Martha and listening to the basement speaker. Osler's words had led me to Beaumont's work and St-Martin's guarded grave, so Osler's answers unsettled me—even our most celebrated physician was obsessed with parts and money—and I knew I would have to look elsewhere. I did not want Martha's family guarding her grave against my exploration. So I wondered whether Martha's dream shake could, alongside Osler's aphorism, give me a clue.

When I became a physician, I learned to see people—friends, neighbors, and strangers alike—as patients. I could see things in them that I could not see before. There were also aspects I could no longer see after I saw people as patients. The most insightful historian of contemporary medicine, Michel Foucault, wrote that medicine was transformed not by creative discoveries, innovative techniques, or the just distribution of resources but when physicians changed how they saw other people.[10] Basement speakers did not discuss these transformations: they acted as if medicine would be transformed by creative discoveries (like Beaumont's deduction of digestion) or innovative techniques or the just distribution of resources. When we talk about healthcare reform, no one talks about vision or perception. Instead they talk about the need for better treatments, better delivery systems, better funding mechanisms.

Healthcare reform is often described as a single event, but in the hospital we experience it as a series of competing initiatives. They overlap in partially coordinated rollouts and launch parties. At one, a policy expert decides that a group of physicians should embrace the patient-centered medical home and hire primary care providers because grants are available to start the program. At the next, a business consultant decides that the number of orthopedists should be doubled to maximize revenue and starts replacing the primary care practitioners with orthopedists. Then a tech guru decides that electronic medical records will increase billing and reduce errors, so he or she persuades the hospital to stop hiring orthopedists or primary care practitioners and spend its capital on technology consults. The changes can be dizzying.

I lack the training to evaluate all these proposals. To do that job well requires decades of training in economics, medicine, public policy, and more. I can offer a participant's view of these changes, of what it is like to live through the reforms celebrated by basement speakers. But my belief is that the best hope for medicine lies in physicians seeing patients as particular, unique individuals—while following, in the words of the Hippocratic Oath, the finest traditions of our calling.

Physicians like me need wise vision to renew medicine. But who can teach us? The basement speaker distrusted wisdom, and now I distrusted Osler. Martha was the only person I had trusted that day, and she had joined the company of the dead. I decided to re-visit my own training to figure out how I had arrived at this place. What lessons in seeing had I already received, and what had they done to me?

two

OCCULT FINDINGS

Osler never autopsied Alexis Bidagan dit St-Martin's famous fistula. The blocked opportunity frustrated him because St-Martin's stomach was the missing piece of the physiological puzzle Beaumont had spent his own life solving. Diagnosis was never completed, Osler taught, until a physician autopsied his former patient, because only the autopsy confirmed or refuted a physician's diagnosis. Osler believed that a physician who autopsied his deceased patients was schooling his vision so that his future diagnoses would be more accurate; *autopsy* literally means to see something with one's eyes, to personally inspect or experience. A physician opened the body of his deceased patient to see for himself how disease traveled through it, how it affected the organs through which it traveled, and where disease eventually accumulated in death.

Physicians are notorious for predicting this path incorrectly. By many estimates, we physicians are wrong about the cause of death as often as we are right. We scribble "pneumonia" as the cause on a death certificate, but when we open the body, the postmortem examination reveals a pulmonary embolism. Knowing this, Osler prescribed autopsies as the best corrective for medical practice. In an 1897 address to the New York Academy of Medicine, Osler advised young physicians to perform autopsies daily, declaring, "Successful knowledge of the infinite variations of disease can only be obtained by a prolonged study of morbid anatomy. While of special value in training the physician in diagnosis, it also enables him to correct his mistakes, and, if he reads the lessons aright, it may serve to keep him humble."[1] Performing autopsies, Osler believed, honed a physician's skill and character.

One of the appeals of reading Osler is that he followed his own prescriptions. He autopsied frequently and learned many lessons from the bodies he explored. By one historian's count, Osler performed 786 autopsies while practicing in Montreal and another 162 while practicing in Philadelphia. Osler grounded his writing and speaking in these autopsies; 160 of his papers are reports of autopsy findings, and he illustrated at least 211 of his public addresses with pathological specimens.[2] Osler believed that autopsies revealed not only the truth of a patient's disease but the measure of the physician-scientist, and he built his career upon postmortem explorations of the body.

Osler was the exemplar of twentieth-century medicine; when Flexner's *Report* was released in 1910, it enshrined autopsies at the center of medical training and practice. In the *Report*, Flexner wrote, "Of . . . essential importance to the rounding out of the medical curriculum is the autopsy-room, where the wise are brought to book," an echo of Osler's conviction that wisdom was obtained by measuring the physician's diagnosis against the book of the disassembled body. Flexner also advised medical students to perform autopsies early in their education, writing, "From an early hour in his pathological work, the student may then begin in the autopsy-room to saturate himself with the clinical spirit." When the *Report* was published, the autopsy rate in the United States was approximately 10 percent; by the 1940s, as American medicine was reformed along Osler's vision, it had climbed to 50 percent.[3]

Although physicians still celebrate Osler's autopsy-honed vision and the reforms of Flexner's *Report*, the autopsy rate in today's hospitals has fallen below even the 10 percent rate Flexner criticized.[4] By the time I began medical school in 2000, I was required to participate in only a single autopsy. It was not enough to teach me how to perform a second autopsy, but it did wake me up to who I was becoming.

• • •

Every ritual has its vestments. For my first autopsy, I went to the medical school cafeteria, then climbed the stairs to the second-floor autopsy suite. Outside the doors, I gowned—I put on hospital-issued scrubs, covered them with a plastic apron, shielded my mouth with a surgical mask, and snapped latex gloves over my hands. Holding my outstretched hands palm up, as if in supplication, I pushed open the door of the dissecting room with my back. As I turned around, I saw an elderly African American man laid out on a stainless-steel table in the middle of the room, his palms open by his sides, his face at ease. He looked kind and paternal, like a sleeping grandfather. He had died hours earlier in the adjoining hospital. Pink puckered suture lines ran up each leg, where the man's hips had been removed and replaced with an alloy of cobalt and chromium. His right foot was blackened and yellowed by diabetes. He was at rest, but the autopsy team was in motion.

A young female pathology resident was my chaperone. As we exchanged greetings, her assistant nodded hello and moved efficiently around the man's body. She asked about my future plans while he opened the man's chest with a single, long incision from the superior aspect of the sternum to the pubis bone. Within five minutes, he was cutting open the rib cage. Within ten, he was examining the organs. He never spoke as he tied off the bowels with kite string, making a long and convoluted sausage that he handed to the resident. She untied it in the sink, spilling out feces as she "ran the bowel," rolling the intestines between her fingers, searching for erosions and fissures and outpouchings, palpating the topographic contours of illness, reading the bowels like a book written in Braille. Despite being up to her elbows in partially digested hospital food, the resident extolled the virtues of pathology as a medical specialty, encouraging me to consider its high-paying, low-hours glory. "And one thing about pathology patients," she joked, "they never miss an appointment."

While we talked at the sink, the assistant remained at the table. He removed the grandfatherly man's lungs, kidneys, heart, and what remained of his gastrointestinal tract and placed them in large bowls, then brought each bowl in turn to the resident. Without comment, she poured each organ onto her cutting board, then sectioned it, her cuts as regularly spaced as those of a bread-slicer machine. After each cut, she inspected the slices for abnormalities, searching for pocketed infections, infarctions, and tumors, exclaiming when she found one. Healthy tissue earned no comment or pause. Meanwhile, her assistant cut the man's scalp from ear to ear, loosened it from the skull, and opened the skull with the oscillating blade of a Stryker bone saw. He drew out the brain for the resident's inspection. She rolled the man's wrinkled gyri between her fingers, looking for signs of abnormal growths or burst blood vessels.

The assistant folded the man's flesh back together, skin sagging over the pillaged abdomen, toweled off some blood, and zipped a vinyl bag shut over his remains. An undertaker would arrive within the hour to fill his abdomen with newspaper and to dress and make the man up so he would be presentable to his kin. The assistant's work done, he left the dissecting room, snapping his gloves into a biohazard waste bin as he left the room.

I was alone with the resident. We stood before a bucket of recently functioning organs, cast aside after her inspection. I asked her whether her work ever led her to consider vegetarianism. "No," she said. "Why would you ask?" There was no use explaining that the grandfather's organs looked like stockyard beef to me. She pushed on, quizzed me about the anatomy of the liver for a few minutes, and then excused me. I left the room and walked downstairs through the cafeteria with no appetite but many questions. How could the pathologist have been so unmoved? She had performed an activity that, in other contexts, would constitute a criminal offense—the dismembering of a body. As I walked home, it occurred to me that one definition of a physician is someone who performs acts so invasive they would be considered assaults if performed outside the physician-patient relationship.

The resident and I were on opposite sides of a division in experience and knowledge, but that gap could be bridged by time and effort. The true division between us was one of perception. As a second-year medical student, I still identified with the patients. When I looked at the man on the table, I saw a grandfather. When the second-year pathology resident looked, she saw body parts. She had learned, as physicians do, to gaze with the eyes of a physician rather than those of a granddaughter, a neighbor, or a friend.

• • •

At the time I attended this autopsy, I was still learning how to see people as a physician does. We were never explicitly taught how to see patients. Our professors did not routinely ask what it means to see or to perceive. They were not art history professors. Medical school professors taught us to see through implicit messages that were all the more powerful because they were delivered by dozens of professors over hundreds of hours of lectures given each morning in windowless lecture halls, reinforced each afternoon in labs, and affirmed each evening in the textbooks we memorized. We reproduced this knowledge during the two or three examinations we underwent each week, mostly multiple-choice tests whose answers we bubbled in on pieces of paper fed into counting devices that turned our tentative answers into percentages. The resulting scores were posted every afternoon outside the rooms in which we conducted our labs. After a few weeks, the test results were papered over one another, like flyers on a telephone pole, the accumulated layers reminding us of all the events we had missed.

After a while, I found it dispiriting to walk into our lab. After all, our experiments were really demonstrations. In our labs we were not testing hypotheses, gathering evidence, or exploring the unknown. We were following procedures our professors had written for us; they knew what should result from our work before we began. The only outcome ever in question was our ability to follow the procedures.

When I began medical school, I presumed I would be trained the way a scientist is. Our exams taught me otherwise. Scientists, like baseball players, are acclaimed if they are successful one of out three times. The grading curve on medical school exams was never that steep. The goal of scientists was to explore; our goal was to consistently replicate existing knowledge. In time, I understood this as apt training for the quality improvement projects of the hospital.

In the moment, I simply understood that I was seeing the body differently. Instead of seeing it as a mystery or a wonder or an embarrassment, I was being taught to see it as a machine. That message was the subtext of every class and lab, but it was clear only in moments that, like the autopsy, forced me to see what I was becoming.

I experienced another of these moments in my first semester of medical school, when I was trying to escape my studies by watching a movie. When the lead actress appeared, I found myself marveling at her clavicle, her body's little key. While watching the movie, I dug into the "bone box" the school had issued to us, a wooden toolbox filled with half of a human skeleton. Some of my fellow medical students were socially clueless enough to carry the bone box with them on the city bus, spooking the other riders by occasionally pulling out a bone to examine the places where ligaments and muscles once attached to its macerated surface. I had thought them weird and overinvested in their studies until I found myself doing the same in the privacy of my own apartment. I suddenly started flipping through textbooks to teach myself that the sternocleidomastoid muscle helped the actress rotate and flex her elegant neck, that the clavicle was the first bone to ossify during development, and that the subclavian vein could be entered by fishing a number 22 needle under the clavicle. As I sat there trying to mimic the insertion of the needle, I realized I was one of the weirdos. A few months earlier, the beauty of the actress's neck would have stunned me. Now I was referencing her to bone boxes and textbooks, reading her body instead of admiring it.

There were other clear moments of self-discovery, moments that seemed designed by Osler himself. In one lecture, we watched a low-budget instructional movie in which a disembodied arm, dissected to expose its bony frame and the muscles that once animated it, was manipulated. Weights were suspended from the major muscles. Each muscle was introduced by the narrator, whose face was not visible in the frame, and then reanimated by a tug upon a weight suspended from a long-stilled ligament or nerve. The biceps would flex or contract, the hypothenar muscles would fold the fourth and fifth digits of the hand into the skinned palm, and we would squirm in our seats.

Upstairs, the glass cases outside our labs were filled with jarred pathological specimens like those Osler had brought to lectures.

On one shelf, you could see embryos at fifteen, sixteen, seventeen, eighteen, nineteen, and twenty weeks' gestation organized in an ascending series like the number chart on the wall of a kindergarten classroom. On another shelf, a collection of hearts lay tagged in the precise spot where they had broken—this one had a transposition of the great vessels, this one was a swollen myxedematous heart, and that one had a *Staphylococcus aureus* infection on the mitral valves. Each specimen had been removed from its context to tell a different story: the transposition told of an embryological defect, the myxedema of an endocrine disorder, and the infection of a substance use disorder. They were parts, pickled in formaldehyde, for us to gaze upon, to recognize by their appearance.

They were also examples of what our own dissections in anatomy class should look like. My first year, we spent two afternoons of every week trying to turn cadavers into specimens suitable for Osler's display. The cadavers occupied the top floor of the medical school; they sat as still in their assigned rooms as we were supposed to be sitting in our lecture rooms five stories below. But if our lecture rooms smelled of a mix of biscuits, coffee, and desire, their rooms had the uniform smell of formaldehyde, the carcinogen that fixed the tissues of the dead so that they would decompose no further.

In groups of four students, we were assigned cadavers as our text for the year. The cadaver I shared was zipped inside a woven nylon bag marked "M" for male, a plastic sheet his only funeral gown. When we unwrapped him, he looked look like a mummy, his ninety-four-year-old body swathed in white hand towels that had absorbed the excess formaldehyde. As we removed the stiffened hand towels, I half expected canned thunder to peal across the room and a hunch-backed assistant to waddle forth. I would have been grateful for the comic relief because what we saw instead was too real for cinema. He lay on his stomach, his face obscured so that we could not develop a relationship with him that might prevent us from using the knives in our hands. The only uncovered portions of his body were the margins, what his lovers might have called his flanks, but which we called the midaxillary line. Our professors handed us scalpels and told us, after a moment's instruction, to cut the back open from the base of the neck to the end of the spine.

That was the second day of med school.

We cut away skin, scooped out fat, and teased apart nerves, ligaments, and muscles to make the dead body before us resemble the copy of Netter's *Atlas of Human Anatomy* we kept beside the dissection table. And we turned the body itself into a book we could read. To do so, we practiced the prerogative of Adam: we renamed limbs, organs, and bodily functions with medical names that were alternately memorial, functional, and structural. The names most likely to stick in my head were the quirky, evocative ones around which I could weave a story. The nodes of Ranvier, the periodic gaps between the myelin sheaths that surround a nerve fiber, made me think of a Frenchman in a cheap beret who latched on to study-abroad students. The anatomical snuffbox, a hollow at the base of the thumb that appears when you extend your thumb, reminded me of an old woman I knew who never went anywhere without a handkerchief and a tin of Tube Rose Sweet Scotch Snuff. The pia mater, the thin fibrous membrane that encircles the spinal cord, reminded me of the medieval hymn "Salve Regina," whose singers seek the mercy of the "tender mother." The more mundane names, the names that described function—like the sternocleidomastoid muscle, whose lateral head attached to the superior border and anterior surface of the medial third of the actress's clavicle—tumbled loosely through my head without ever quite lodging themselves into a viable sequence. On the cadaver floor of the med school (what would have been called the Dead House in Osler's day), I followed the course of this nerve or that ligament with difficulty, struggling to find the through line that would reveal nature's design, but not to confirm any diagnoses or prior knowledge of the body. Instead, this was our inauguration into a physician-patient relationship like the one Beaumont had with St-Martin.

Our days of tedious work were punctuated by outright butchery. After we learned what we could from, say, the skin of the thigh, we would break out large-toothed handsaws and cut off the legs of our cadaver in savage movements, one classmate bearing down hard on the blade and another pulling down on the soon-to-be-severed limb. In one of these moments, a classmate, a future orthopedic surgeon, asked, without irony, "Don't you just feel better with a knife in your hand?"

Only a little. Holding the knife between my thumb and middle finger, my index finger directing the blade from above, I was the dissector rather than the dissected, a tremendous relief, but I never felt the surge of purpose my classmate felt with a scalpel in his hands.

We would occasionally lay down our scalpels in favor of a cartilage knife, a dissecting forceps, or a probe. No matter which tool we used, our dissection felt remote from science. The results of the dissection did not matter. We would not discover a new organ. The relevant outcome was our transformation from student to physician. We students were being marked off from our future patients by virtue of our knowledge, experience, and most of all our perception. By cutting the legs off a cadaver, we were inducted into the club of people who spend their lives being intimate with the bodies of strangers. We saw sights others did not see and performed activities others did not undertake.

At this same time, one of my sisters was training to be a nurse. She told me that during her first week she learned to make a bed so her patient would be comfortable. I told her that I had hacked away at the muscles of an old man's back to make them look like the picture in a textbook. The difference between the formative experiences of our professions seemed clear. She would tend to the body, I would take it apart.

• • •

I now know that physicians, nurses, and all the other people who work in hospitals and clinics can be dispassionate and empathetic by turn. And yet I remember those distinctions in my training and my sister's because our different formations taught us to see people in different ways. My sister was trained to see an ill person as someone needing succor. I was trained to see an ill person's pathology.

As Osler's children, we physicians are taught to see the body by looking at the dead. That is what startled me about becoming a med student. Instead of admiring the arching beauty of an actress's neck, I was observing the prominence of her clavicle and wondering how best to slip a needle beneath its inferior surface. Instead of making a bed for a dying man, I was scissoring, sawing, and sculpting his flesh into a version of the diagram in my textbook. Instead of saying good-bye to a grandfather who had just died, I was helping a pathologist read his bowels. The way I saw the body was changing.

When you read histories of medicine, you learn that this is by design. Osler was at the apogee of a movement that began in the late eighteenth century, as physicians started combining their practical experience with scientific knowledge gained from dissecting bodies. Before this, medicine was largely pattern recognition and the exercise of clinical judgment. Dissection occurred, of course, but even famed anatomists like Galen dissected animals instead of humans. Medical students did not routinely dissect. Instead, a student aspiring to be a physician apprenticed himself to a senior physician and, after some unstandardized period of time, began practicing independently. Medicine was local and personal, and the results were wildly inconsistent. To improve them, physicians needed a reliable body of knowledge, and they gained that knowledge through dissection. Physicians abandoned centuries of taboos about invading the body of the dead, taboos still held by families like Alexis Bidagan dit St-Martin's. Physicians violated these taboos so they could identify diseases that were previously hidden from view. I could feel the weight of those taboos—Do not disturb the rest of the dead—as I removed leathered skin, tweezed stilled nerves, and chiseled calcified bones.

We broke these taboos in search of what we could not see from the intact body. In medicine, we call concealed signs of disease "occult findings." We do not mean that they are evidence of the supernatural or mystical, but that they are secret, obscured from our view, and, by implication, that all such things should be brought into our view.

Medicine was transformed when physicians learned to see *where* they could not previously see, inside the body, and *what* they could

35

not previously see, internal pathology. In 1801, Marie-François-Xavier Bichat, a French physician reared in a previous form of medicine not united to anatomy, told his colleagues, "For twenty years, from morning to night, you have taken notes at patients' bedsides on affections of the heart, the lungs, and the gastric viscera, and all is confusion for you in the symptoms which, refusing to yield up their meaning, offer you a succession of incoherent phenomena." He advised, "Open up a few corpses: you will dissipate at once the darkness that observation alone could not dissipate."[5] Physicians were being taught that a body yields its meaning only through dissection, not through the life, labor, and love a person undertakes with it.

I read Bichat's words in Michel Foucault's *Birth of the Clinic*, in which Foucault described the moment when physicians combined dissection with clinical practice as the "great break in the history of Western medicine."[6] Instead of seeing themselves as people designated by society to attend to people who are suffering, they began to think of themselves as scientists. We now understand ourselves as people who observe and measure the body, hypothesize about its function and dysfunction, and then prove and disprove the resulting theories. When physicians began understanding themselves as scientists they developed antibiotics, anesthesia, and antisepsis. With these disruptive and innovative technologies, they transformed what it means to care for the ill. They also transformed themselves.

• • •

Many physicians remain committed to perceiving themselves as scientist-humanists like Osler. He was the great teacher, beloved by his students. Just as he cared about his students, he cared intensely for his patients. He read widely, taught often, and practiced constantly. By most accounts, Osler was the ideal. He saw much and he saw wisely.

I worry, however, about the adverse effects of accepting Osler as the ideal to which physicians should aspire. If Osler is the ideal physician, then the ideal patient may be a corpse. After all, even though Osler was an internist, Osler reformed medicine by placing pathology at the foundation of clinical medicine. He declared pathology to be the proving ground of a physician's skill and character, even though it teaches us to see the body as a collection of diseased parts, a decidedly incomplete view.

To his credit, Osler died as he lived, following the advice he gave to others by sanctioning a postmortem dissection. At his request, Osler's autopsy was carried out in his home, on the day after his death at the age of seventy. The dissecting physician removed Osler's brain, then examined the remaining organs. He confirmed many of the diagnoses made during the great physician's final days but was unable to determine the source of the hemorrhage that killed Osler. The book of Osler's body did not reveal a definitive cause of death. Five days after his death, Osler's body was cremated, the ashes eventually interred as a relic at his memorial library.

But one part of Osler's body was not cremated. Osler had donated his brain for study. A paper was eventually published that crudely, but favorably, compared Osler's brain to those of other dead scholars. The authors concluded that what made the great physician great was observable to the trained eye in the size and shape of the gyri and sulci of his brain. After the research was completed, Osler's brain was relegated to a formaldehyde-filled jar. Parts of his brain went missing over the years—clippings from the pages of the great physician— but they were eventually tracked down, purchased, and placed back in the jar. Now the brain of Osler lives on as pathological specimen at a research institute in Philadelphia, his most famed part achieving the fate he sought for St-Martin's fistula.

Some gifts are really warnings. In our first month of medical school, we received two such gifts when the University of North Carolina, like medical schools around the world, held its white coat ceremony.

If dissection was our private induction to medicine, the ceremony was our public one. The first took place in a windowless lab at the medical school, the second in an august auditorium on the main quad of the campus. It was held on a weekend. Parents came. Pictures were taken. Punch was served. Parting gifts were passed out: a book and a coat, white, as promised.

The coat was an emblem of our noble calling. It was placed over our shoulders, stiff and untailored, still bearing the creases from its packaging. We knew that as we tended to people who were bleeding or vomiting or otherwise making a mess on us, the coat would receive the stains of our experiences. We also knew that we were expected, somehow, to preserve its whiteness. When the coat got dirty, we were to clean it. When we could no longer bleach and starch it into a semblance of its original state, we were to replace it. As a gift, the white coat implicitly warned us to maintain a distance from the ill. The coat was to mark us out from other people.

The book, *On Doctoring*, was an anthology of texts about practicing medicine. Every year, each American medical student receives a copy. It is, in all likelihood, the only book all American medical students own. It includes essays, poems, and stories—a miscellany of love letters about being a physician.

The book and the coat: ritual objects, one might think, handed down to medical students since the time of Hippocrates. In fact, the book, the coat, and the ritual at which we received them are all recent inventions of the humanism-in-medicine movement, whose aim is to reform medicine by encouraging students and physicians to take a more humanistic approach to medicine.

The association of the white coat with physicians can be traced back to the era of William Osler. In his own clinical practice, Osler favored a full suit, but he wore a white apron when dissecting, and he would have understood the impulse behind the white coat, which makes physicians resemble laboratory scientists. The association was intentional: when Osler began his career, physicians were only one group among many types of healers jockeying for public approval. Many physicians were poorly trained patent medicine peddlers competing for patients with local homeopaths, hypnotists, and hydrotherapists. Osler helped physicians distinguish themselves from these other healers by teaching them to present themselves as scientists, who, at the time, often wore tan lab coats to protect their clothes during experiments. Lab coats were practical and without pretense. In the late nineteenth century, many surgeons adopted the light-colored lab coats in the operating theater to signify their commitment to the new, antiseptic techniques. These surgeons were clean; their coats were the proof.

The physicians' lab coats also made their wearers look like priestly counterparts of the nuns who staffed many nineteenth-century hospitals. Like a priest's robes, the white lab coat suggested the purity and power of its wearer. By the time Osler died, the white lab coat was widely associated with physicians. They were scientists. They were professionals, deserving their authority and society's respect.[1]

By the time of my training, the white coat was so essential to the physician's public presentation that we acquired two of them in the first month of medical school, one at the ceremony and one purchased, unceremoniously, from the medical school bookstore. Practically, we preferred the second coat, because we wore it to protect our clothes while we dissected cadavers. These were work coats that no patient would ever see, so they could have been any color, and yet none of my classmates purchased anything other than a white coat. Politically, we wanted a white coat because it signified our status as medical students. In a tan or blue coat we might have been confused with the janitorial staff. We were training to be physicians, so we selected white coats for the privilege they conveyed. We kept these coats on the top floor of the medical school in closets outside the dissecting rooms, where they soaked up the potent chemicals. By the semester's end, they were so damp that they clung to us like primer on fresh boards.

The honorary white coat was startlingly clean and emitted the sugared smell of perchloroethylene and other dry-cleaning solvents. It was cut short at the waist, to indicate our place in the medical hierarchy. Senior physicians wore long cotton coats with braided buttons. Resident physicians wore long polyester-cotton-blend coats with translucent buttons, their names embroidered over the heart. Intern physicians also wore long poly-cotton-blend coats, but with the name of the hospital stitched where they hoped their own name would someday reside. Our short coats had neither name nor logo.

At our white coat ceremony, Dr. Stewart Rogers, a respected internist on the faculty, addressed us. He described the white coat as a symbol representing the "Mantle of Hippocrates." So far, so traditional: we were going to invoke the great physicians of old and claim a bright line connecting us back to them. Then Dr. Rogers asked whether we would wear the coat as apron or as armor.

Armor would protect us, and Dr. Rogers admitted that we would need protecting. The white coat, he told us, would help us "stay clean and calm—for the next patient, for our families, for our peace of mind." The coat would even help us maintain enough professional distance to avoid burnout. The coat, he hoped, could protect us while preserving our empathy.

But he cautioned that we would eventually need that empathy, and he clarified: "The white coat is an apron, not a suit of armor, and you'll appreciate the design—it opens over your heart." The coat opened over our hearts to allow our empathetic engagement with patients. He observed that a white coat would show stains, and warned us, "Never forget that the worst stains spill from your own character: from neglect, impatience, or greed." He noted that the coat could also serve as a satchel for the tools we carried and as a badge of our clinical privilege. He advised us to feel gratitude to the citizens of our state, who generously subsidized our education. He urged us to appreciate the "creativity, conscience, humor, kindness, generosity, or courage" of our patients. Finally, he concluded, "There is also a warning, in fine print, that some of you may forget to read: 'This coat will fit better and last longer if you do not wear it all the time.' Remarkable as it is, your white coat will not exhaust all your talents or meet all your needs. So hang it up sometimes, even during medical school."[2]

It was a bracing speech. Dr. Rogers had delivered real advice. Be grateful for the coat. Be worthy of the coat. Be afraid of the coat. He is the first physician I remember sounding a warning about what medicine could do to its practitioners. And I was struck by how personal his warning was. He did not talk, like many of the people I knew, about disliking his job or his boss. He talked about fearing what being a physician did to him and what it could do to us.

His words seemed to dissipate quickly, however: We were here to celebrate. Who was this old man issuing warnings? We were wearing party clothes. Why was he hanging crepe? The remaining speakers offered aspirational exhortations. They called us to the elevated stage, enrobed us in white coats, and welcomed us to the profession. We recited the Hippocratic Oath. The audience cheered. The auditorium cleared, but Dr. Roger's warning stayed with me.

Walking home, I did not feel as though I belonged to the profession. I still identified with the patients, not the physicians. Although I left the ceremony with a truncated version of an attending physician's coat, I felt like a fraud. I was not a junior physician, half as good as a practicing physician, but a mere student. If I dropped out of med school during the next month—and a couple of my classmates did—I could tell people only that I used to be in med school, not that I used to be a physician. If I wore the anonymous white coat outside the hospital, I would look much more like a busboy than a physician. But when I wore the coat in the hospital or clinic, I received an undeserved share of the physician's privilege. A week later, when I told Gloria's son that she was dead, the coat added professional privilege to the list of privileges—those of race and class—that divided us.

Years later, certain objects would make me feel like a real physician—a pager, a prescription pad, my first student loan bill—but not my anonymous white coat. Part of the reason for this was because the day's ritual seemed forced, like a concocted religious service. Most of the audience were dressed in their Sunday best, and we sat together in a sanctuary, listening to inspiring words, but the ecstatic moment never arrived. I heard the warning issued by Dr. Rogers in his remarkable homily, but the ritual never provided the release I expected. The ritual felt like a stage show. As, in fact, it was.

• • •

The white coat ceremony dates only to 1993, when it was first performed at Columbia University through the sponsorship of the Arnold P. Gold Foundation. Named after its founder, a renowned child neurologist on the Columbia faculty, the Gold Foundation sponsors research, awards grants, and introduces initiatives such as the white coat ceremony to promote humanism in the medical profession.

Gold and his wife, the generous sponsors of these initiatives, are seeking to reclaim what they believe has been lost in medical education and practice. When Gold compared his own training to that of a contemporary medical student, he saw it as both more demanding and more humane. When he described apprenticing himself to a Dr. Smith, for example, he wrote, "I slept, ate, and stayed at the side of my patients. Dr. Smith's behavior was my curricula; her values informed my own. There were none of the competing values and messages that are prevalent today. Residents and students did what their attendings modeled. Altruism was the rule, and meeting the needs of the patients, whatever the personal cost, was the norm."[3] He regretted that in contemporary medicine this apprenticeship model and its values have been eroded. He wished to restore the synthesis, personified by Osler, of rigorous science and empathetic humanism in medical education and practice.

Gold wrote that he developed the white coat ceremony at Columbia "to welcome new students into the profession and introduce them to their responsibilities toward patients."[4] These responsibilities chiefly include virtues like compassion and humility. As Gold described it, each ceremony has a common structure. Students are welcomed to the profession of medicine, they recite an oath of their choosing, are cloaked in white coats, listen to an inspiring address by a leading physician, and then celebrate at a reception. The Gold Foundation actively supports the adoption of the ceremony, offering grants to pay for a school's first ceremony if the school will commit to future ones. The ceremony has been adopted by the majority of American medical schools, as well as by medical schools in countries as far-flung as Australia, Germany, Pakistan, and the United Kingdom; it has also been adapted for pharmacy and physician-assistant schools.

The white coat ceremony has become a ritualized induction of medical students into the profession, but it is also an effort to renew the practice of medicine through Osler-style humanism. The foundation is always expanding its scope: it operates the Gold Humanism Honor Society to recognize medical students, trainees, and physicians who exhibit clinical excellence and humanistic care; it recently announced that it planned to design a parallel ceremony for resident physicians as they begin their training; and it sponsors professorships for faculty members engaged in encouraging humanism in medicine. The foundation's goal is for every physician to be a humane physician. I admire the Golds, their foundation, and their earnest work, but the ceremony unsettled me. Dr. Rogers's warning—that it was the defects in our character that would most stain our white coats— seemed a more fitting induction than the ceremony itself.

I am not alone in feeling discomfited by the ceremony. Some observers fear that the ritual reinforces the hierarchies of medicine.[5] Unlike nursing students, who wear surgical scrubs during training, medical students wear dress clothes underneath their white coats, marking themselves as white-collar professionals. As students in our short coats, we were on the bottom rung, but we were on the professional ladder, and the ceremony made me want to ascend the ladder, to be worthy of the long white coat. The ceremony encouraged our solidarity with the profession, not with our future patients, and signaled that we were members of the medical profession, with a measure of its associated responsibilities, to be sure, but also with a measure of its privileges. As long as I was wearing the white coat, no one would ask why a medical student a month into his training was watching Gloria die and then telling her son about it afterward.

The ceremony also communicated to us that professionalism and humanism were equivalent. The professional student physician was the humane student physician. In an essay explaining the ceremony, Gold wrote that "humanism is the central aspect of professionalism," as if humanism were a part of professionalism, rather than a separate but related concept.[6] In Gold's writings and the work of his foundation, the words *humanism* and *professionalism* are often used synonymously, as they were, to my surprise, at the ceremony. I had always understood humanism to mean being oriented toward rationally addressing the needs and well-being of a person, and in the context of medicine, it seemed to me that humanism meant putting the needs of the ill person, or patient, first. I took professionalism to mean possessing or displaying the skill and character of a member of a particular profession. In medicine, it seemed as though professionalism meant aspiring to be like Osler, a skilled and respected physician. If the foundation really wanted to emphasize humanism, why not give medical students a gift that reminded them of their solidarity with the ill rather than their identification with physicians? Or, since our short white coats resembled those of busboys, why not tell us that we were the servants of our patients? Why not have us pledge something like the Oath of Maimonides, in which an aspiring physician promises to "never see anything in the patient but a fellow creature in pain?"[7] Or why not omit oaths altogether? A recent survey found that only one in four practicing physicians describes medical school oaths as influencing his or her current practice.[8] Our ceremony was well-intentioned, but it collapsed the differences between serving the needs of patients and fulfilling the responsibilities of the profession.

Dr. Rogers discussed the white coat's multiplicity of uses—armor, apron, satchel, and badge—and warned us about the potential cost of wearing it. But the ceremony insisted it had only one use: it was "the mantle of our profession." In celebrating the coat as an ancient symbol, it obscured its history as a modern invention, part of the shift toward conceiving physicians as scientists.

• • •

Every religious community needs sacred texts. At our white coat ceremony, the dean of the medical school passed out copies of the *On Doctoring* anthology as ours. We carried them home in our white coats, although they were quickly replaced in our pockets by practical, instrumental texts with miniscule type and more diagrams and tables than paragraphs. In an era before smartphones, most medical students carried a trio of pocket books—the *Maxwell Quick Medical Reference Guide*, the *Tarascon Pocket Pharmacopeia*, and the *Sanford Guide to Antimicrobial Therapy*. There was barely a metaphor among them, let alone a poem or story. So the anthology seemed like a real gift, bound in hardcover, and protected with a dust jacket. On the dust jacket was a reproduction of Norman Rockwell's 1958 *Saturday Evening Post* painting "Before the Shot," in which a white-haired, white-coated physician is preparing to administer an injection to a young boy. The physician's skin is also white, as was that of most of the writers featured inside the book—certifiably great, capital A authors such as Auden, Chekhov, and Hemingway.

The era depicted by the Rockwell painting represents the pinnacle of physician authority in America, and the whole book had a wistful quality to it. Back then, it suggested, physicians were well compensated, well respected, and well obeyed. The book's contents were engaging but reverential, as if medical training and practice were comparable to a series of Rockwell scenes in which the physician was a central character. The texts did not reflect the usually disjointed, occasionally hilarious, and often tragic experience of medical training and practice. When the dissenting voices in the anthology criticized physicians, it was to describe someone who did not live up to the standards of the profession, not to question the enterprise of contemporary medicine. Most of the excerpts contained an easily extractable moral lesson.

The texts seemed to have been selected and excerpted in order to make Osler happy, even if, as far as I can tell, none of them came from Osler's reading list. Osler liked writers from an earlier canon. He loved Cervantes, Emerson, Epictetus, Montaigne, and Plutarch.[9] None of these authors appeared in *On Doctoring*. And there were other differences. Osler recommended a small library of books to his students, often the entire corpus of a writer. We received a single book. Although Osler loved books about medicine, his reading list covered a broad range of topics. We received only texts about physicians. Still, there were continuities between Osler's reading list and the anthology. Most important was the humanistic tone of the texts. In addition, readers were encouraged to identify with physicians rather than patients. The experiences of the authors, many of them physicians themselves, provided a further link. Osler had called the graduating army surgeons out of their own communities and into the community of physicians, and the anthology was implicitly doing the same. Even though the authors and the texts had changed from Osler's day, this book was, like the white coat, an updated version of Osler's reform. Physicians were to be scientists and humanists.

Like the white coat, the anthology was paid for by a foundation interested in renewing the practice of medicine in the manner personified by Osler. In 1989, the Robert Wood Johnson Foundation created it with a stated goal of altering the tone of medical education and practice, and has subsequently paid for each American medical student to receive a copy.

Although the effect of the anthology on contemporary practice would be hard to assess, it is difficult to overstate the role that the Robert Wood Johnson Foundation plays in contemporary medicine. Through its Clinical Scholars Program, the foundation has trained two generations of leaders in academic medicine. The foundation is the largest American philanthropic institution dedicated specifically to healthcare, and it distributes around $400 million in grants annually. In this context, the *On Doctoring* anthology is a small but tangible symbol of the foundation's philanthropic portfolio and its efforts to alter health and healthcare.

For me, it would be hard to say that the anthology altered my life. I read it once but found it relentlessly uplifting; a few months later, I included it in a box of books that I took to the used bookstore. They offered me only a dollar in store credit for the anthology. When I asked why, they pointed to a shelf of five other copies and said, "Med students drop them off every year." I traded the anthology for one of the books excerpted in it, Abraham Verghese's memoir *My Own Country*.

Recently I started thinking about the anthology again and wondered why a large philanthropic organization would take pains to fund and distribute it. In one of the Robert Wood Johnson Foundation's published reports, the anthology's editors, Richard C. Reynolds and John Stone, described the book's genesis. As a high school student, Reynolds had read Sinclair Lewis's *Arrowsmith* and A. J. Cronin's *The Citadel*, early-twentieth-century novels with idealistic physician protagonists directly inspired by the Oslerian reform of medicine. Reynolds wrote that the novels sparked his interest in medicine. When he joined the foundation staff in 1987, he also recalled an initiative by the pharmaceutical company Eli Lilly that from 1923 to 1953 paid for every graduating American medical student to receive a copy of *Aequanimitas*, a collection of Osler's speeches. Reynolds remembered this as a happier moment, when pharmaceutical companies passed out books rather than advertisements to physicians. He recalled asking representatives of the industry earlier in his career if they might distribute classic medical texts, including Beaumont's account of dissecting Alexis St-Martin—a reference I found telling. The goal of the anthologists was truly Oslerian.[10] They, like Osler, wanted physicians to read Beaumont's writings on gastric physiology, implicitly encouraging students to identify with other physicians rather than with patients like St-Martin. The anthology was implicitly teaching medical students how to listen to the stories of the ill. The anthologist wanted me to listen to those stories so well that I could, in my own practice of medicine, craft each patient encounter as confidently as the authors in the anthology. The aim was to keep idealistic medical students from becoming alienated physicians by teaching them to attend closely to their patients by reading, and even writing, empathetic literature. The anthologists wanted me to be the expert reader, or maybe even the author, of the people I would meet as patients. That seemed to me like a good way to promote professionalism, but if we want to encourage medical students to embrace humanism, perhaps they should instead be asked to read a patient's account of being ill and receiving medical care—the story told from St-Martin's perspective rather than Beaumont's.

In joining professionalism with humanism, the anthologists continued the work of Osler, who believed medical humanism to be as essential to reforming medicine as autopsies. He pressed a standard reading list upon his students and trainees. He quoted great literature in his talks—in his address "The Army Surgeon," in which he encouraged the graduating physicians to see much and to see wisely, Osler managed to reference Thomas Browne, Thomas Carlyle, William Shakespeare, Laurence Sterne, and Hebrew Scripture. Osler understood himself within a tradition of Anglo-Saxon writers and spoke to his trainees as if they belonged to the same tradition. So when Osler told the graduating army surgeons—"Your praise shall still find room. Even in the eyes of all posterity"—he was using a Shakespearean love sonnet to laud his audience.[11] Medicine was a humane science that was ever progressing, its practitioners were heroic, and literature from great white English writers offered the proof. In addresses like the "The Army Surgeon," Osler, like the *On Doctoring* anthology after him, obscured the particularities and the histories of the texts he cited in order to narrate stories of the humane physician as a constant throughout Western history.

• • •

The conflicting messages about professionalism and humanism in the white coat ritual established a pattern for the rest of medical school. Moments of hard-earned wisdom were obscured by the constancy of professional formation. Our formal education was often truly humanistic. Our medical school employed a department of scholars in social medicine who introduced students to the economics, ethics, and history of medicine and scores of learned clinicians who impressed upon us the need to be humane in our care of the ill. These clinicians taught me what I did not know when I saw Gloria die: how to speak with and examine patients. Every Wednesday afternoon, we had formal lessons to learn how to talk like a physician. My teacher was a family physician named Donald Spencer. When you meet a patient, he said, "You introduce yourself. You ask their name. You ask how you can help them." Dr. Spencer made it seem natural. He moved about an exam room with poise and purpose. His face defaulted to a smile. When he spoke, his voice was soft but certain. Patients were reassured. Students were inspired. He spoke of the responsibilities we had to our patients.

I heard him.

I admired him.

Yet on my clinical rotations I learned something different—how to see people as compendiums of parts and money. When residents and attendings quizzed me about a patient, they never asked about his or her strengths or passions; they wanted to know about the physical exam findings, lab values, and pathophysiology. When no one asks about something, you learn that it is not important. Medical educators call these kinds of formative learning experiences the "hidden curriculum" or the "null curriculum," which contains the implicit messages that medical students receive in training through what is not discussed. The hidden and null curricula undo the work of the Dr. Spencers of the world.

As I came to the realization that Osler's grand synthesis, the first contemporary proposal to reform medicine, confused professionalism and humanism, I began to remember many examples from my training. When I was a third-year medical student, I received a community service award for volunteering at the medical school's free community clinic, where we provided check-ups, screenings, and referrals for people who could not afford medical care. For me, the work was a reminder that many people cannot afford healthcare and a chance to offer a bit of service. The award was a hardbound copy of the same anatomy atlas we had used when dissecting cadavers as first-year students. Today this prize copy of the atlas sits on my office shelf—its pages clean and spine intact. It is a sanitized version of the book I once used in the cadaver lab, with pages oil-stained by human fat and paperback binding broken in thirteen places. The prize copy seems to represent a sanitized version of my training, something that obscures the messy history of medical training and practice. Although I appreciate the award, I prefer objects whose history is more apparent and acknowledged.

I still own a white coat. I am an attending physician now, so it is a long white coat. It is made of cotton, and its buttons are braided. Dr. Rogers observed that our white coats opened over our hearts to allow us to engage our patients empathetically. That is a statement of humanism, but on the coat I own, my name and title are embroidered over my heart. My professional identity is announced over the metaphorical home of my empathy. On my coat, as often occurs in medical practice, humanism loses out to professionalism.

Still, I remembered Dr. Rogers's warning, and I eventually heeded it. As a medical student and resident, I wore a white coat constantly, but I no longer wear it very often. It resides on a hanger in my office, unstained but dusty.

I have not, however, stopped searching books for thoughts on how best to be a physician, so I recently read the book passed out to a previous generation of physicians, Osler's *Aequanimitas*. The title refers to the professional characteristic of, as Osler writes, maintaining "a calm equanimity" in the face of any situation. "The Army Surgeon" is included in *Aequanimitas*. So is an address from 1901, "Books and Men," in which Osler remarked, "It is hard for me to speak of the value of libraries in terms which would not seem exaggerated. Books have been my delight these thirty years, and from them I have received incalculable benefits. To study the phenomena of disease without books is to sail an uncharted sea, while to study books without patients is not to go to sea at all."[12] I was struck by his metaphor: the physician as ship's captain, setting out on a sea of illness, with books as his charts and guide. I wondered whether it might point me to a version of humanism in medicine that did not collapse into mere professionalism.

I decided to reread some of the books that had guided me in medical training, beginning with the book for which I traded in *On Doctoring*, Abraham Verghese's *My Own Country*. I remembered the book's humanism and wanted to see whether it could still inspire me on my search as I set out on the seas Osler had charted for us.

Sometimes a book finds you at the right time. I felt that way when I first read *My Own Country: A Doctor's Story*. It was the second year of medical school, and I was feeling discouraged. I saw the book on the shelf of a classmate I admired; she said it had motivated her to become an infectious disease physician. I needed motivation, so when I saw a yellowed copy at the used bookstore, I picked it up.

I started reading it that night. The author, Abraham Verghese, wrote with impressive fluency and apparent passion. Verghese was a disheartened physician, but he still professed nothing but love for examining patients and teaching students. I quickly fell under his spell. In fact, all of medicine soon did as well, and Verghese became a leading physician-writer. Over the next two decades, Verghese developed an Osler-style proposal for renewing medicine through reading literature and carefully performing physical examinations, a proposal that began in the pages of *My Own Country*. So I reread it recently. For the second time, it was the right book at the right time. This time, I realized that the memoir's peculiar magic is that it portrays a physician as the storyteller of his patients' bodies, taking something like full responsibility for telling his patients' stories.

My Own Country focuses on Verghese's first job in the long white coat of an attending physician. Before taking the job, Verghese was an infectious disease fellow in Boston, a city renowned for its academic medical centers. As a fellow, Verghese had learned that infectious disease physicians could, with careful diagnosis and targeted treatment, cure people of their infections. After completing his fellowship, Verghese moved to Johnson City, Tennessee, a place removed from renown. About the same time, the AIDS epidemic arrived in Johnson City, and since there were as yet no effective treatments for the disease, Verghese found that he could care for his patients, but he could not cure them. In moving to Johnson City, Verghese was living out Osler's advice to the army surgeons. He had accepted a posting to a remote locale, with rural Appalachia substituting for Osler's army outposts on the colonial frontier, and he made the most of it. As the only physician caring for persons with HIV and AIDS in the area, Verghese saw much. He rose before dawn to make rounds at the hospital, then slipped away to his laboratory to research pneumonia, and spent his afternoons seeing patients in an infectious disease clinic, where he became the primary physician for a group of people with HIV who had been shunned by the local physicians. After clinic ended, he often attended advocacy meetings or made house calls instead of returning home to his wife and young children. Verghese admitted that his work caused tension with his wife, but he could see no other way to be the kind of physician his patients deserved.

The book had everything the *On Doctoring* anthologists could wish for—the protagonist was reflective, the writing fluid, the message humanistic, the subject topical—while it endorsed the kind of work ethic every residency training director wants in his or her residents. Verghese was no critic of medicine; he was, rather, a disappointed idealist, whose highest compliment was that a colleague was "a careful and thorough physician."[1] I could see why his book was selected for the anthology; it instilled a useful hope in me.

Verghese's hope for the renewal of medicine was that physicians would return to the bedside and personally engage patients through a physical examination. He wrote, "I loved bedside medicine, the art of mining the patient's body for clues to disease. I loved introducing medical students to the thrill of the examination of the human body, guiding their hands to feel a liver, to percuss the stony dull note of fluid that had accumulated in the lung."[2] His descriptions of his patients were articulate and precise, if clinical, and as he shaped their stories, he portrayed physicians as the expert readers of the body, people who read the body like a familiar text.

To Verghese, the paradigmatic act a physician performs is to read the body through the physical exam, but the pleasure of being a physician lies in teaching trainees how to do the same. Verghese celebrated everything about the Oslerian teaching service—the authoritative examination, the detailed presentation, the learned discussion—and in this sense *My Own Country* was the perfect book for a medical student. It made my training, and my place at the bottom of Osler's ladder, seem purposeful. I was learning to be the same kind of humane and skilled physician that Verghese became through his own training. If I followed the plan, I too would ascend the hierarchy of the teaching service. I too would become a humane physician.

But Verghese also alerted me to what would happen if I did not follow the plan. Throughout his memoir, he criticized peers for performing careless and perfunctory physical examinations. He lamented that most contemporary physicians aspire to be exquisite technicians who perform specialized procedures with consistency and speed without engaging their patients. Since those procedures were much better reimbursed than bedside medicine, cardiologists and surgeons earned more money than infectious disease physicians like Verghese, and their higher income accorded them greater status among medical students, hospital administrators, and their neighbors. Verghese faulted healthcare's financial hierarchy for discouraging humane encounters with patients.

I welcomed this kind of justification during my preclinical years, when I spent most of my days being examined or lectured to. My work seemed absurdly distant from the goal of caring for real people. Reading Verghese gave me the hope that if I submitted myself to the seemingly pointless rituals of medical school, I would become something approximating the physician Verghese described.

Verghese also gave me hope that I could be a good physician by attending carefully to the body through the physical examination, organizing signs and symptoms into revealing clues. When you rolled up sleeves to take a patient's blood pressure and found raised purple patches, they signified Kaposi's sarcoma, and when they were accompanied by symptoms like fatigue and weight loss, they suggested an

HIV infection; such signs and symptoms could be organized into a compelling story. As the physician in a remote region, Verghese told these stories, stories of particular ill bodies but also of a group of "prodigal sons," young men who grew up closeted in rural Appalachia, left to live openly as gay men in urban centers, contracted HIV/AIDS, and returned home to die.[3] Their stories were powerful medical science and humane literature.

I aspired to be such a physician and writer, so I appropriated Verghese's commitment to internal medicine along with his frustrations about procedural medicine and his hopes for the renewal of medicine. The hope I borrowed from Verghese helped me through the preclinical years of medical school. I endured lectures and exams while waiting for the third year, when the clinical training would begin. When the day arrived, I was eager for the hospital and gratified to be assigned a teacher who reminded me of Verghese. Dr. Samuel Cykert could describe the results of dozens of studies and the efficacy of hundreds of medications from memory.

He ran his hospital service according to the Oslerian rhythm. We students would arrive before dawn, gather data, and then pass it along to the residents, who corrected and organized the data into presentations. When Dr. Cykert arrived, we would make rounds. We examined the patient's parts in order, from head to toe, and then by rank, students first, then the interns, the residents, and the chief resident. Afterward, Cykert would complete the portions of the exam we had missed. Together, we percussed the liver searching for dull sounds, flashed penlights in pupils to assess for light reflexes, and listened to lung fields for whispered pectoriloquy which could indicate to the ears of an experienced physician the presence of cancer or pneumonia. Then Cykert would ask a student to name the finding, assemble a differential diagnosis, and venture a treatment plan. He questioned, or "pimped," the student until he or she reached the end of his or her knowledge. Then he would move hierarchically through the rest of the group, asking more difficult questions of the intern, then the resident, and finally the chief resident. When the knowledge of the entire group had been exhausted, a rhetorical space would have been created out of the gaps in our knowledge, and within that space Cykert would teach us, filling in those gaps. Cykert pimped us mercilessly. I feared his questions because they revealed my ignorance, but they also inspired me. I wanted to understand my patients so well that I could answer Cykert's questions. It was a worthy goal, but it also meant that every patient became a test, an opportunity to assess my own ability and worth.

My chance to prove myself came late one afternoon when I admitted a young man who reminded me of Verghese's prodigal sons. Demetrius was a thirty-two-year-old gay man who had returned to his mother's house two months earlier. He was thin and colorless, like a picture book faded by the sun, and his mother thought it odd that, even in the thick heat of a southern summer, he wore long sleeves to cover his arms. But she looked the other way because her son was home, whatever the reason, after a decade away. When he did not come downstairs one morning to pick at his breakfast, she opened his bedroom door and found him unconscious on top of sheets stained with blood.

When his ambulance arrived at the hospital, he was already receiving his second liter of normal saline through an eighteen-gauge intravenous needle. The Emergency Department nurses and physicians stabilized him, but it was clear that he could not return home, so they paged the admitting team, Cykert's team. We were on call, responsible for following the patients already admitted and for admitting new patients overnight. It was early in the afternoon, and there was still time for teaching, so the resident encouraged me to take the lead.

I pulled back the curtains surrounding Demetrius's bed and conducted the history and physical exam. He would start a conversation and then, overcome by fatigue, lose the thread and fall silent. Meanwhile, the resident physicians wrote orders to admit Demetrius to the hospital. It took them five minutes to write the orders. It took me two hours to complete my assessment, because I was determined to stitch together the right story, to assess Demetrius in a way that would pass Cykert's examination while being as articulate as one of

Verghese's stories. Even as I examined Demetrius, I was startled by the way his experience resonated with Verghese's memoir—the patient had identified as gay from a young age but remained closeted until he left his rural North Carolina hometown for Washington, D.C., where he lived openly as a gay man, contracted HIV and hepatitis C, buried his partner, and then, in grief, stopped the antiretroviral medications that checked his infection. Over the previous year the infection had progressed until he could no longer work, so he had returned to his mother's attic to die. He told me all this as I percussed his liver, auscultated his lungs, and examined his eyes. I evaluated him in between interruptions for more urgent interventions: phlebotomists drew blood, nurses hung additional bags of saline, and aides cleaned his periodic bouts of bloody vomitus.

When Demetrius was transported to the intensive care unit, I organized my notes into a story. We paged Cykert, and I presented Demetrius to him.

"The patient is a thirty-two-year-old male with HIV, CD4 count unknown, and HepC brought in by ambulance with hypotension."

Cykert interrupted. "How low was the BP?"

I shuffled through my notes. "97/64."

"Go on."

" . . . and vomiting blood."

"What blood type?"

"Um, not sure."

"Find out. Go on."

So I went on. On and on, Cykert stopping me at every one of my many mistakes. Finally, the chief resident came to my aid, telling us we were being paged to examine Demetrius on the floor. As we walked, Cykert told me to correct the presentation. He examined Demetrius in three minutes, efficiently resolving all the questions my presentation left unanswered. He suggested a few changes to our orders and went home.

I spent the night at the nurse's station in the ICU, writing and rewriting my presentation. I hunted through the unit's tattered copies of *Harrison's Principles of Internal Medicine* and the *Washington Manual of Medical Therapeutics* for clues on how to improve my presentation. Again and again, I rewrote the presentation, but it never seemed Cykert-worthy. I could not get the story right, and I began to perceive my situation as desperate.

Fifteen feet away, Demetrius was experiencing a truer kind of desperation. He was still bleeding. He had esophageal varices, pathologically dilated veins, from the blood backing up from his faltering liver. His varices loosened, and with every beat of Demetrius's heart, blood leaked into his esophagus. The nurses hung bag after bag of blood—it was O positive—throughout the night. A visiting gastroenterologist fellow threaded an endoscope through the burbling blood, looking for a place to cinch up a varix band or inject a clotting agent. She could not find one. She called in the attending gastroenterologist from home. Bleary-eyed, but with experienced hands, he fared no better. Meanwhile, the nurses kept hanging bags of fluids and medicines until Demetrius was surrounded on either side by IV poles that were propping him up.

When Cykert returned early the next morning, I presented the patient again. There were no interruptions this time. While Cykert sipped his cup of coffee, his experienced eyes scanned the unit. Halfway through my presentation, Demetrius vomited blood again. Cykert walked briskly into Demetrius's room, the group following. Receiving no answer to the questions he posed to Demetrius, Cykert called the code, the hospital-wide announcement that a patient was in mortal distress. The unit awoke in unison. Physicians, nurses, and respiratory therapists worked to save the dying prodigal.

They all failed. Demetrius died a frantic death, alone in a crowd. I felt dispirited, both for my patient, the second person whose moment of death I had witnessed, and for my hopes of becoming a particular kind of physician. Verghese had convinced me that the physical examination, the performance and presentation of it, would allow me to see the patients before me clearly, to be present to them in their suffering. Instead, I had spent Demetrius's dying hours trying to write the best description of his body.

I never read Verghese the same way after that night.

• • •

Verghese published another memoir and then a novel, but I did not read them. They were not the right books for those moments in my life. Then, a few years ago, my inbox started filling up with essays, op-eds, and commencement speeches written by Verghese. Physicians who were frustrated with the practice of medicine were passing around these writings like samizdat. I received them, often with subject lines imploring me to "READ THIS!," from former classmates and from our hospital's chief medical officer.

When I did so, I was reminded of the appeal of Verghese's writing. He wrote well and cited great literature with medical themes. He diagnosed the ills of medicine. He prescribed a treatment.

In his medical journal essays, Verghese wrote for his fellow physicians, sharing his regrets that technology now dominates the field of medicine. Verghese lamented that instead of attending to a patient at his or her bedside, we attend to technological abstractions of a patient, the electronic medical record or the lab values or imaging studies.

I sympathize with his complaint. Most days, I spend more time documenting patient care than being with my patients. I wonder how much more I could learn about patients if I spent my days with them instead of their charts. As an attending, I frequently tell medical students and residents to ignore their smartphones while speaking with a patient, only to find myself distractedly looking at my own electronic minders. Even when we spend more of our time with our patients, even when we put away our devices, we often pay more attention to a patient's blood work than to the body from which the blood was drawn.

Verghese understands this, and like Osler he recommends reading certain texts. Unlike Osler, he specifies literary fiction with medical themes. Verghese advises physicians that such texts can help them understand their patients through the literary tools of narrative, character, and metaphor. This advice appeals to me; I read constantly and find that narratives offer me a way to understand my life and the lives of the people I meet as patients. Verghese, however, extends the argument, asking physicians not just to read the tale, but to become the teller. When he spoke to a national gathering of internists a few years ago, he argued that physicians could renew medicine by understanding themselves as "storytellers, storymakers, and players in the greatest drama of all: the story of our patients' lives as well as our own."[4] For Verghese, these kinds of close readings refocus the physician on the patient.

Verghese believes that the physical exam also leads to such refocusing. He discourages physicians from performing the kind of cursory physical examination I watched on my first day with Gloria's rural physician: The doctor spends a few moments assessing what he or she suspects will be the diseased parts of a patient's body, then checks "WNL," an abbreviation for "within normal limits," in the medical record. In such cases, the doctor may never know what he or she missed. (Privately, physicians joke that "WNL" actually means "we never looked.") Verghese wants more physicians to be like him and Dr. Cykert, and like Osler before them—careful performers of the physical examination. To this end, Verghese, now a professor at Stanford, and his colleagues have developed the Stanford 25, a list of twenty-five physical examination techniques they teach to students, trainees, and attending physicians. They are offering not only a diagnosis and prescription for contemporary medicine but also a compelling hope: that physicians can renew medicine if they refocus their attention on the individual patient through the physical examination. This diagnosis, prescription, and hope are captured in the slogan of the Stanford 25: "An initiative to revive the culture of bedside medicine."

• • •

So what happens when a physician practices medicine in this fashion, when he or she stays at the bedside to read the diseased body and tell its story? It was when I had progressed in my medical training and started thinking more deeply about this question and the larger questions of how we see our patients that I returned to *My Own Country*. Much of the memoir still inspires, because Verghese rendered the suffering of his patients as compelling case histories of men and women infected with a virus that stigmatized them before it killed them. Since no cure was available, Verghese learned to care for his patients with HIV/AIDS by carefully attending to them. In doing so, Verghese developed a clear hope that attending carefully to what the body has to tell will allow a physician to see the suffering person on the hospital bed clearly, and thus become a "good" physician. But *My Own Country* also transmits an implicit warning. While rereading it, I found passages inappropriate for our aspirational anthology, passages where the light fades fast. These sections show the alienation Verghese experienced through the stigma of AIDS, the loneliness he felt as an outsider in Appalachia, the strains his work inflicted upon his marriage, his anger at the greater pay and social status afforded physicians who perform procedures instead of sitting with patients, and most of all the difficulty of facing his patients' deaths.

Toward the end of the book these tensions culminate at the bedside of Luther, a man with AIDS whom Verghese knows well. Luther has been hospitalized, and Verghese is examining him, accompanied by a full teaching team. He usually describes examinations of patients with students and trainees as his happiest moments, but in this instance he is annoyed with the students for being more impressed by "numbers from a Swan-Ganz cardiac catheter" than by the physical examination of a patient. Their attention is consumed by technological abstractions. Verghese ultimately faces his own limitations at Luther's bedside:

> The medical students and residents are quiet, hovering around the bed, uncomfortable because death is staring at them. I am uncomfortable too, and I am angry all the time now. This is what I think when I lie awake at night: I want to start all over again. . . . When I began in Johnson City, I was ambitious, fascinated by the [HIV] virus and by my patients. I maintained no distance, denying to myself that this was a fatal illness. The future, when all my patients were dying, seemed remote and vague. I convinced myself that I could handle that. But I simply did not understand how devastating it would be to watch. All the stories that I have painfully collected have come to haunt me with

their tragic ending, as if I am the author and must take full responsibility. In a new place I can begin again from a wiser and more careful vantage. The students and residents are waiting on me. I have been lost in thought. What am I supposed to do here, at this bedside?[5]

I was startled by this passage. As a practicing physician, I now know how devastating it is to know someone, care for that person, and then watch the person die. The truth about medicine is not that some patients die despite our efforts but that every patient eventually does so. What I missed when I read this passage as a student was that part of the anguish for Verghese was that he had made sense of a dying person's suffering through his own actions. As Verghese put it, the physician can become, in a moment like this, an author who "must take full responsibility" for the deaths of his patients. By accepting that responsibility, Verghese crossed the line between reader and writer, and he felt as though he had in some way created Luther's body and brought about Luther's death. Under the weight of such responsibility, Verghese fantasized about quitting his job, leaving the state, and starting over. In the moment, though, he remained at Luther's bedside, surrounded by students waiting, like children eager for a bedtime story, for him to read the text of this dying person to them. Was he the reader or the author of the text? What was a physician to do, here at the deathbed?

For Verghese, the answer was clear. In his next line he wrote, "I have, for which I will always be thankful, the ritual of the examination." He put his hand on Luther and examined his dying patient. Although Verghese insightfully asked what physicians were supposed to do at the deathbeds of patients like Luther, the answer he offered in his memoir, the answer he has repeatedly offered over the ensuing two decades, is that they should return to the ritual of the physical examination. And yet a physical examination is surely, like the numbers from a Swan-Ganz catheter and the reports in the electronic medical record, an abstraction of the body, albeit in a different degree. In each instance, a physician takes on the responsibility of interpreting the meaning of a patient's body, a responsibility that can stagger even our most skilled physicians.

And what about Luther? What solace could he take from being expertly examined, from being read well, by a physician and his trainees? I do not know, and Verghese provided me with only an indirect answer. In *My Own Country*, Verghese wrote that a physician's diagnostic power, which made a patient visible to the physician, allowed him to interpret seemingly unrelated signs and symptoms as part of a single disease. By naming signs and symptoms as disease, a physician could reduce the stigma experienced by many of his patients. Many of Verghese's patients with AIDS were shunned by friends and family; what a relief it must have been to meet a physician who would see and touch them despite their illness.

However, by seeing them in the manner he did, Verghese also took on a fearsome responsibility. In his memoir, he tabulated the cost of undertaking such intimate readings of his dying patients. These responsibilities so alienated him from himself, his family, and his work that he did ultimately leave Johnson City. Rereading Verghese's memoir at a later stage in my own career, I clarified the misgivings about his prescriptions that I had experienced at Demetrius's death: his proposal to renew medicine advocates seeing much because it reinforces the role of physicians in contemporary life as *the* people with full responsibility for reading and interpreting the body, for determining its meaning.

There are, of course, humane proposals to renew medicine that do not place full responsibility on physicians. Some shift the authority in a physician-patient relationship entirely to patients or their caregivers. Some propose reviving medicine by engaging humane disciplines—art, history, literature, music—other than science.

Most of the medical humanities proposals that, like Verghese's, are embraced by healthcare practitioners, adopted by medical schools, and circulated over email by physicians are not so radical. They represent what the physician Jeffrey Bishop calls the "dose effect" of humanities, the idea that we ought to "give medicine and medical students a dose of humanities so that medicine can become (once again?) humanistic."[6] Many of the most popular dosing regimens, like the white coat and the anthologized book of wisdom, subsume humanism into professionalism. At the hospitals at which I have trained and worked, one of the most popular proposals along these lines is Schwartz Center Rounds.

Schwartz Center Rounds are funded by the Schwartz Center for Compassionate Healthcare. The center's inviting motto, "Join us in Transforming Medicine," indicates the scope of its goals. It wants to renew medicine by increasing compassionate care for patients, a move that it believes will reduce burnout among care providers. Schwartz Rounds began at Massachusetts General Hospital in 1997 but now take place regularly at hundreds of hospitals across the country. Schwartz Rounds are confidential, multidisciplinary gatherings in which physicians, nurses, and other healthcare professionals reflect on the burdens, challenges, and gifts of caring for the ill. The meetings, usually occurring over lunch in a hospital auditorium, are open to practitioners but not to patients and their families. They typically begin with a narrative summary of a case and are followed by an open discussion of how it felt to participate in the case. In an article reviewing a decade of Schwartz Rounds at Massachusetts General Hospital, the oncologist Richard T. Penson and his colleagues observed that Schwartz Rounds were very well received, writing, "Caregivers yearn for an opportunity to express themselves openly in a situation in which it is safe to do so and . . . they derive great benefit from the feedback and support they receive from colleagues."[7] As Penson suggested, Schwartz Rounds are designed to offer a place where caregivers can express themselves, in order to relieve the weight of full responsibility placed upon them by contemporary medicine.

When I first attended Schwartz Rounds, I did experience the relief that comes from sharing a burden to which one had become accustomed, but there was also a surprising feeling of familiarity. It felt like grand rounds, the weekly lunchtime meetings in hospital auditoriums where members of a clinical department gather to discuss a difficult case and listen to an eminent physician share the latest research associated with the patient's condition. As in grand rounds, senior practitioners usually framed the conversation. As in grand rounds, practitioners at Schwartz Rounds told stories about patients in order to teach a lesson. As in grand rounds, practitioners at Schwartz Rounds discussed, rather than engaged with, patients. In both settings, the patient's story is told by practitioners for the edification of practitioners. As Penson wrote, "The Rounds focus on caregivers' experiences, and encourage staff to share insights, own their vulnerabilities, and support each other."[8] I appreciated the relief, but Schwartz Rounds struck me as something much less than the transformation of medicine. Later, when I read more about Schwartz Rounds, I saw that the Schwartz Center understands them as the humane version of grand rounds; the familiarity I experienced is intentional.

At least part of the success of Schwartz Rounds is due to that familiarity for medical practitioners who are already accustomed to learning Osler-style lessons from the bodies of patients. It was Sir William himself who popularized the grand rounds tradition while teaching at Johns Hopkins. I could not escape the great physician and his influence; he kept showing up unexpectedly. In the Schwartz Rounds, it was the use of patient stories for the education of practitioners. Even when the message was quite different—I find it impossible to imagine a contemporary Schwartz Round speaker advocating for coerced autopsies—the form is the same. Physicians see much, therefore we see wisely. In Osler's model, and in the model of the medical humanists like Verghese who followed him, the physician determines the meaning of an illness. We now see quotidian events of human existence—conception, childbirth, adolescence, pregnancy, old age, death—as events in which a physician should intervene. Even the proposals, like the Stanford 25 and the Schwartz Rounds, that set humanism at the heart of medicine do not unseat physicians from their place as the people with something approaching full responsibility for interpreting the body.

We may be able to renew medicine through stories, because we all make meaning through stories, but we will not do so if the stories are told by physicians for the use of other physicians, if we continue to imagine physicians as having full responsibility for their patients' bodies and lives. Perhaps the solution lies in the opposite direction—preventing physicians from taking on full responsibility by regulating the bodies and time of physicians themselves.

Drug dealers gave up using pagers years ago, but we physicians still clip them to our belts or to the reinforced pockets of our white coats. Some female physicians slip them inside the collar of their boots, where the small black box resembles the electronic monitors that parolees wear to track their movements.

We use pagers because they are an inexpensive way to track the members of a medical team as they disperse across the warrens of a contemporary hospital. While we are on call, we send each other pages to remind ourselves which patients to revisit, what results to follow, when to admit new patients, and where to catch lunch. When a pager emits one of seven preprogrammed tunes from its tinny speaker, we all reach for our belts to see who has been called. Pagers that frequently go off are known as "dirty bombs" because they act like shrapnel, disrupting schedules and plans. When a shift ends, we quickly pass our pagers off to the next physician.

There is one pager you cannot pass off: your personal pager, the number at which you can always be reached, no matter where you are working or with whom. The personal pager represents one way the body of a physician is regulated in professional responsibilities.

• • •

Everyone agrees that physicians are professionals. We have obligations to patients that go beyond simply doing whatever we can do for a patient or doing what a patient requests us to do. We are obliged to uphold the ethical and technical standards of medicine. Humanism and professionalism may often be confused with each other, but professionalism is worth pursuing in its own right. We know that students who engage in unprofessional behavior are more likely to become physicians who engage in behavior that harms patients, so some efforts to renew medicine are aimed at fostering professionalism among students, trainees, and practicing physicians.

One effort is "Medical Professionalism in the New Millennium," a physician charter produced by leading American and European medical organizations. The charter identifies three principles—patient welfare, patient autonomy, and social justice—and expands them into ten commitments.[1] The commitments are all reasonable—engaging in lifelong learning, being honest with patients, maintaining patient confidentiality, respecting appropriate boundaries, improving the quality of care, increasing access to care, pursuing cost-effective care, appropriately using science and technology, avoiding conflicts of interest, and self-policing the profession—but toothless. The principles are abstract. The commitments are nonbinding. Few physicians even realize that their professional organizations have committed to these principles on their behalf.

The charter is an aspirational consensus statement, one of many statements and studies, centers and curricula, ideas and initiatives aimed at bolstering or inculcating professionalism among physicians. All are well intentioned. Most of them, like the charter, are concerned with the ways physicians can regulate their own behavior.

Yet none of these initiatives are as influential as the practices that regulate the time and movement of physicians. A physician can choose to engage with or ignore a charter but must respond to the systems that govern his or her time. For the past couple of decades, pagers have symbolized the kinds of governance that enforce a physician's professional obligations.

As a medical student, I carried pagers for a series of teams named after the parts of the body for which the team cared. Hematologists. Thoracic surgeons. Pediatric cardiologists. Gynecologists. Neurologists. I joined each team for a prescribed period of time. Two weeks with the urologists. Four weeks with the oncologists. When I joined each team, I was always asked the same three questions: name, rank, and pager number. Then someone would quickly introduce everyone else on the team by name, rank, and pager number. It was like the nerd version of the meet-up scene in a war movie where a new infantry unit is assembled from the remains of several others.

When I first joined these clinical teams as a third-year med student, I figured myself for a future internist or surgeon, a physician with dramatizable skills. Internists were mapmakers, mapping patient symptoms and diagnostic test results onto unseen organs within the body, deducing what was going on inside the body without disturbing the skins. Surgeons were explorers: distrusting maps of unseen locales, they parted the veils of skin and fat to gaze directly upon diseased tissue or aberrant structures, then removed or repaired them.

As the third-year student, though, I had few skills beyond fetching coffee, charting fever curves, and debriding wounds of necrotic tissue. My job was to fit myself to the team, to pattern my actions on the members'. They approved of me when I imitated their actions. They disapproved of me when I asked why we engaged in those actions. Surgeons disliked questions on rounds because questions kept us from the battlefield of the operating room.

On the surgical team, my pager and I were assigned to a pair of towering interns. The first had a gap-toothed smile and bushy hair parted at the left; despite his hair, everyone called him Gandhi because he was so coolheaded and even-keeled. The second had short, tightly curled hair cut close to his scalp, glasses too small for his face, and perfect teeth; we called him Cannon.

Cannon never learned my name, preferring to call me Rookie, or just Rook, as if I were the PFC to his second lieutenant.

Cannon was unhappy with his place on the ladder. He had wanted to enroll at an American medical school but wound up at an international school instead. He had wanted to specialize in orthopedics but had settled for general surgery. He had hoped to train at a private hospital but wound up at a state-sponsored school where, as he ruefully noted, there were "lots of poor folks on these wards, Rook."

Our first shift together, he promised to show me "how medicine works." We made rounds before dawn, wrote notes through lunch, visited the operating room in the afternoon, and spent the evening admitting patients from the Emergency Department. Our schedule was frequently altered when more urgent concerns were brought to our attention by our pagers.

Around three in the morning, a nurse paged us about one of our team's postoperative patients. The patient had intractable hiccups that kept her from sleeping.

I summarized the concern and asked Cannon, "What should we do for the hiccupping lady?"

"Tell the nurse hiccups are *not* a surgical problem."

"But it's our patient."

"Okay, Rook, look up the treatments for intractable hiccups."

I opened the computer, searched online for the treatments, and read them aloud, "Chlorpromazine. Haloperidol. Methylphenidate. Baclofen. Midazolam. Rectal massage."

"What was that last one?"

"Rectal massage."

"Uh-huh. That's the one. Rook, let me teach you. You've got to show the nurse who is in charge. Call them and tell them we want PRN rectal massage to treat those hiccups."

"No way."

"Wuss. I'll call."

Cannon did. The nurses were angry, but he insisted. Rectal massages every fifteen minutes until the hiccups remitted. Doctor's orders. The nurses massaged the patient's rectum for the rest of the night, and for the next half-decade every nurse in the hospital made sure to page Cannon mercilessly every time he was on call. Cannon did not sleep much in residency, but he did teach me something about how medicine worked.

Up all night with surgical and medical services as a student, I was awed by their knowledge and exhausted by their work ethic, but realized that I did not belong on either team. I began to worry that I fit into no service at all.

When I started on the psychiatry service, I was dismissive, believing that it was not real medicine. I scheduled the rotation for December because I had already scheduled my wedding for January. My future wife, Elin, and I were classmates. We heard that psychiatry was a less demanding rotation than some others and figured it would give us time to finish our wedding preparations. I expected to be as uninterested in the work as I was in selecting flower arrangements. Instead, I found myself treating a drifter who walked around town with a backpack full of rocks because he believed that gravity had lost its hold on him. I met a sleepless young woman who filled pages of a notebook with equations purporting to show how the lyrics of pop songs reconciled classical and quantum mechanics. I met an addict whose drug of choice was Sanka per rectum. I found a team that offered what I liked best about medicine and surgery. Like internists, they deduced illness without disturbing the skin. Like surgeons, they addressed once-hidden issues. But psychiatrists were less interested in mapping illness or exploring pathology for their own sakes than in helping people learn to live with their individual realities. During those six weeks of psychiatry, I realized where I belonged. I married Elin and decided, to my surprise, that I was going to be a shrink.

When I finished the rest of my rotations, I enlisted in North Carolina's psychiatry residency and traded my short white coat for the longer, but still anonymous, white coat of an intern. I was ascending Osler's ladder. My first name receded from conversations, replaced by "Doctor," and I started to carry the call pager.

On the second night of my internship, an exhausted colleague handed me the pager for the first time. She chuckled while shuffling out to the parking lot at the end of her thirty-hour shift. As she drove away, I realized that I was the last physician standing, the only on-call physician for a large state mental hospital named after its founder, the nineteenth-century social reformer Dorothea Dix. At its peak in the 1970s, the grounds of Dix Hospital unfolded over 2,354 acres that included three lakes, a working farm, a cemetery for deceased patients, and 282 buildings housing 2,756 patients. By the time I arrived, most of the acreage had been sold to developers, and most of the patients had been turned out onto the streets. In its diminished state, Dix resembled a failed nation-state, overgrown with stands of long-leaf pines, its remaining buildings falling back into the earth. Some buildings housed adolescent boys who yelled all night, others old men who slept all day. Some buildings sheltered women who plucked unseen bugs from the air, others girls who cut their legs open in red, ragged stripes. All told, the hospital accommodated up to 600 patients and was staffed by 1,300 administrators, cooks, custodians, nurses, physicians, and technicians.[2]

Most of these personnel worked during the day. At night, a few nurses staffed each unit. Their chief job was to keep the nights quiet, but nights were rarely quiet for the only physician in the building, the on-call intern. When I was on call, the nurses would page me for a sleep aid to silence a manic talker or an antipsychotic pill to pacify a paranoid mind. I welcomed the calls I could resolve with a one-time order for clonazepam or risperidone. I feared the calls that required me, no matter the hour or the weather, to drive across the dark hospital grounds to see a patient in person.

On those nights, the pockets of my white coat would be crammed full. In addition to a stethoscope, pocket manuals, and pens, I carried car keys, so I could move from building to building, and unit keys, so I could unlock the doors when I arrived. When I pushed through the heavy steel doors, their windows woven with steel wire, I could often hear the patient I had been paged to examine. If not, the nurses would direct me to a naked child smearing his feces inside a seclusion room or a crying woman banging her fists against an unbreakable window. My job was to speak with the staff about what had occurred, attempt to reason with the patient, write a note documenting the incident, and leave behind orders for medications. On those call nights I saw much more than it seemed a person should, witnessing these low moments in harshly lit rooms with aged linoleum floors that bore crude traces of all the other low moments that had come before. The work left its own traces on me.

I saw much and learned much at Dix. How to start intravenous fluids on a person who cannot keep still. How to distinguish a heart attack from a panic attack in a person who cannot speak coherently. But I also learned: Keep your distance. Offer only real choices. Make modest promises. Address only the most urgent matters now and put off to the morning everything else. Keep a checklist of everything you promised to do. Sleep when you can. Answer the pager when the admissions office calls.

The admissions office at Dix was located in the main building, next to the loading dock. Ambulances and police cruisers from across the state would back into the loading dock and release their cargo into the waiting room. One of the three admissions workers would check a patient in, while another would call my pager.

"You've got another patient."

"Another?"

"Yes."

"Okay, I'm over in the adolescent building checking out a bite. Little vampires. Then I promised the forensics unit I would assess a guy with the shakes. After that, I will be heading to . . . "

"You need to come now, this guy's out of control."

The admitting patients, like the forward guard of an attacking army, rose to the top of any checklist. There were no nurses in the admissions office, so I had to leave the bitten adolescents and the tremulous prisoners for later in the evening. Driving back across the grounds, the cemetery where unclaimed bodies were buried on my left, I arrived at the main hospital, where the admissions workers greeted each patient from behind a windowed wall. After they finished, I met each patient in an adjacent room, sitting if it seemed safe, standing near the door if it did not. I worked alone, becoming faster, if more facile, as the training progressed. What had taken me two hours as a student took me fifteen minutes by the end of residency. Working those night shifts, I learned to efficiently and effectively introduce myself, engage a patient, obtain a history, perform an examination, and develop a treatment plan. I developed instincts. I started to feel the rhythm of an examination, to know when I was sounding a false note and how to regain the rhythm when it faltered.

In all of this, Osler was proving to be right. My repeated, constant experiences in a rural outpost were training my vision, widening it until I could see much. I became a physician capable of admitting five, ten, fifteen, even twenty patients in a single shift, all while responding to emergencies on the rest of the campus.

But though I was becoming experienced, I was not becoming wise. Indeed, to get through the shifts, I learned to divide my attention. I cut patients off after I had heard enough of their story to complete my admission note. I learned to placate instead of listen.

I also learned to pinch myself on the wrist when I felt myself falling asleep. As fatigue enveloped me, I would be unable to stop my frustrations from leaking out. I would become short with the nurses. I began avoiding eye contact with patients and became more Cannon-like with every call. Ashamed by my behavior but exhausted by the demands, I retreated into myself, hiding out in the call room whenever I could. The room was furnished with castoff furniture: a lamp without a lightbulb, a bed with a rubber mattress manufactured during the Carter administration, a desk whose top was occupied by a television that received four channels when the weather was clear, a disposable telephone borrowed from a better hospital, five-year-old magazines whose glossiest pages were cemented together, takeout menus. The windows had been bricked in to allow for sleep whenever sleep was available. The room had its own toilet and sink, and a shower shared with the hospital's spiders. Still, I would sit alone in the call room whenever I could, savoring moments of quiet. If time allowed, I would eat a greasy delivery dinner alone. An attending physician was available if I needed assistance, but he or she was always a phone call away, sleeping at home. When I did call the attending, he or she often sounded annoyed—I was an unpleasant reminder of their own experiences as a resident. I called the attending infrequently, but the frequency of calls to pager seemed to increase as the night progressed. By the early hours of the morning, as the calls escalated, my behavior had eroded. My questions grew shorter. My responses were reduced to grunts and nods.

But I held it together until early one morning I found the limits of my equanimity. A patient was in a diabetic crisis, and I had requested help that was not yet available. The patient's nurse disliked the delay, so he "hammer paged" me every thirty seconds, demanding that I discontinue my orders for frequent blood draws. I explained my rationale, promised to search for another solution, and pleaded with him to stop paging me. All to no avail. He paged again and again, yelling at me each time I called back. Finally, I threw the pager across the call room, experiencing a frisson of delight as it shattered. Silence. Freedom from the professional minder. In the newfound quiet, I could see that dawn would soon arrive, and not longer after, sign-out.

Even the most dramatic nights ended with sign-out, at which I handed the pager over to the day team. Then I would return to the call room, shower, prop myself up with coffee pilfered from the nurse's station, and go back upstairs to see my regularly assigned patients. When I finished that routine, I would escape to the parking lot, still wearing my white coat over hospital-issued scrubs. On the drive home, I listened to sports talk radio because the arguments kept me awake without involving me emotionally. I kept my hands on the wheel and tried not to hit anyone.

Or to hurt anybody at home. I shared a home with Elin and our two-year-old, Eamon. Elin and I were both on call every fourth night, so we staggered our nights so that one of us would always be home. We saw each other mostly in passing that year. One day, napping after a call night, I awoke to the sound of the front door. I went to check and found that Eamon had climbed out of his crib, opened the front door, and started toddling toward the street. I raced out of the house in my underwear, scooped him up, and locked the door behind us, wondering how the three of us would survive Osler's residency curriculum.

• • •

Osler had been named the chief physician of the newly founded Johns Hopkins Hospital in 1888; by 1890, he and the rest of the Hopkins faculty were calling their trainees "residents" because the trainees resided at the hospital.[3] By the 1900s, the American Medical Association was publishing lists of approved residencies. In these

75

residencies, trainees would work every day and every other night. By midcentury, resident physicians were working thirty-six-hour shifts every other day, more than a hundred hours a week.

A typical example of this work ethic was endorsed by one of Osler's protégés, Dr. Rufus Cole, in a commencement address to the graduating medical students at Cornell University in 1938. Cole began his speech by summarizing the sorry state of medicine before Flexner's *Report*. Then he celebrated the transformation of medicine into a science in the years after Flexner. Through their schooling, Cole said, medical students acquired scientific understanding, but upon graduation they were not yet ready to practice medicine. They needed to acquire practical skills, and the only way to do this was "by practice itself and by unremitting hard labor" in a hospital.[4]

Since some internships were just open-ended visitations in which a recent medical school graduate spent as long at the hospital as he (most graduates at the time were men) felt necessary, Cole advised the graduates to seek internships in which trainees lived in the hospital as residents. "During your intern days, the hospital should be your home, your workshop and your playground. You should need nothing more. Learn to shun outside affairs that will complicate your life and disturb concentration on your work, rejoice if you are too poor to own an automobile to carry you from the straight road, avoid the movies, you will find sufficient tragedy as well as comedy close at hand, above all, avoid like a plague entangling affairs of the heart."[5] This was the kind of advice the protégés of Osler frequently gave. Work hard. See much. Avoid life outside the hospital. Stay away from movie theaters.

By the time I trained, the Oslerian model was still considered the ideal, but it was running up against new realities. Thanks to advances in medicine and changing criteria for hospitalization, the average patient in the modern hospital was more ill than during Osler's era and required greater attention. The length of hospital stays was shorter. The expense of medical training and education had increased. In addition, medical school classes were now evenly split between men and women, making affairs of the heart harder to avoid.

For me, it was far too late to avoid them. Elin and I were committed to medicine, but we did not want the hospital to be anything more than a workshop. We did not need the hospital to be home or playground. We shared a home and lived near an actual playground, where our son delighted in the swings, his legs knifing through the humid air. Watching Eamon was a joy and a glimpse at an alternative model of care—instead of the quick fixes and crisis responses that we were learning in the hospital, our son was teaching us the accretive work of parenting.

Our playground visits were less frequent than he would have liked. To have enough money to pay for our son's daycare, I often picked up extra, moonlighting, weekend shifts at Dix. Many evenings, we felt lucky if we could collect Eamon from his daycare before someone called social services, share a meal together, read a bit from a textbook or journal article after he went to sleep, and then find our way to our own bed. Cole had no reason to fear we would waste our training at the movies. But was this system truly the way to produce competent and caring physicians?

In March 1984, at a hospital affiliated with Cornell, the medical school where Cole had given his commencement speech urging "unremitting hard labor" a half-century earlier, an eighteen-year-old named Libby Zion died while her own physicians were half-awake. According to an account by the writer Natalie Robins, *The Girl Who Died Twice*, Zion was admitted to the Emergency Room with symptoms of agitation, fever, and flulike complaints. When physicians evaluated Zion, they could not piece these symptoms together into a compelling diagnosis and misdiagnosed a "viral syndrome with hysterical symptoms."[6] Zion's physicians that evening, a first-year intern and a second-year resident, were working long shifts. They admitted her to the floor and ordered intravenous fluids and acetaminophen. Zion remained agitated, swearing and pulling out her intravenous lines; the resident ordered meperdine and, later, haloperidol. Then, while the resident retreated to an apartment across the street from the hospital for some furtive sleep, the intern worked her way around the hospital, seeing other patients while answering pages. Zion's nurses paged the intern twice that night, concerned because Zion remained agitated and awake. The intern ordered that Zion be placed in a restraining vest. Zion finally fell asleep while the intern kept moving, working through her checklist. When a nurse checked on Zion later in the morning, she was running a high fever and could not be roused. And then her heart stopped. Libby Zion died less than a day after being admitted to the hospital.

An autopsy was ordered, but the results shed little light on Zion's death. It wasn't until years later that a consensus was reached that the biological cause of Zion's death was serotonin syndrome, a rare adverse medication reaction. Before she arrived at the hospital, Zion had probably been using cocaine and marijuana, along with the prescribed drugs chlorpheniramine, diazepam, erythromycin, flurazepam, oxycodone, and phenelzine. Phenelzine is a nonselective and irreversible monoamine oxidase inhibitor that can effectively reduce depressive symptoms but is often difficult to tolerate. When a person ingests phenelzine, it prevents several neurotransmitters—dopamine, epinephrine, melatonin, norepinephrine, and serotonin—from being degraded, so more of these neurotransmitters are active in the body. It also, however, prevents the degradation of tyramine, a component of fermented foods, smoked meats, many cheeses, and most alcohols. Ingesting these foods while taking a drug like phenelzine can result in a dangerous elevation of blood pressure.

Taking phenelzine and cocaine in combination with meperdine, a synthetic opiate better known by the trade name Demerol, and haloperidol, a dopamine-blocking agent that is commonly used to reduce agitation, can also lead to dangerous, even lethal, levels of serotonin. As serotonin increases in the body, the person can become agitated and tremulous, experience diarrhea and a fever, begin to sweat or shiver. Each of these symptoms can be caused by thousands of diseases, so piecing them together into a single diagnosis, serotonin syndrome, is challenging. Zion's physicians were not up to the challenge. I suspect I would not have been either.

Errors occur often in the hospital. I remember being on call once when a resident ordered ten times the usual dose of a furosemide, a diuretic, for a patient. The patient received the dose before the resident realized her mistake. The resident immediately disclosed the error to the patient, the patient's family, our attending physician, and the hospital. The resident was disconsolate, but the patient's family said they understood. The family remained understanding even when the patient died the next day. The patient was elderly, and the family felt that she had made her peace with dying.

Zion's family was not so forgiving; their daughter was only eighteen years old. Zion's father, an attorney and journalist, subsequently dedicated his life to correcting the kind of error that led to her death. But what exactly was the error? Was it that Zion had received fragmented medical care both outside the hospital, where she received medications from her college's physicians along with her home dentist, gynecologist, pediatrician, and psychiatrist, and inside the hospital, where at least five separate physicians were involved in her care in the space of eight hours? Was it that the patient did not disclose her illicit substance use and her prescription drug misuse to the admitting physicians? Was it that the resident physicians missed a difficult diagnosis? Was it that the hospital lacked pharmacy safeguards to prevent the administration of medications that could cause serotonin syndrome? Was it that the resident physicians were insufficiently supervised by attending physicians? All these factors seem relevant to the tragic death of Libby Zion.

But Zion's family concluded that the error was the "unremitting hard labor"—the long duty hours—of the residents on call. They launched a crusade that led first New York State, in 1999, and then all accredited American residencies, in 2003, to limit a resident's workweek to eighty hours and shifts to no more than thirty hours. In 2007, the United States Congress asked the Institute of Medicine to explore the association between medical errors and resident work hours. In its 2008 report, the institute recommended that, whereas a resident's workweek could extend up to eighty hours, an intern shift should last no more than sixteen; that residents working thirty hours should have at least five hours nap time; and that moonlighting should be discouraged.[7] In 2011, the Accreditation Council for

Graduate Medical Education (ACGME), which accredits most of the eighty-five hundred or so American medical training programs, implemented an even stricter version of these rules. A trainee can now work up to eighty hours a week, but interns can only work up to sixteen-hour shifts and residents only up to twenty-four-hour shifts.[8] The surprising outcome, though, is that while today's trainees may theoretically have more time to catch a movie, their shifts have become even more demanding.

In this century, Osler's training model has been transmuted from in-house residencies into high-pressure shift work. Far from living in the hospital, today's residents come and go constantly. They are issued pagers, but most prefer to use their own smartphones, devices that even more precisely track their comings and goings. They need to keep track, because they arrive and depart at prescribed times, sometimes literally being sent home in the midst of caring for a patient because they have reached the end of their allowed duty hours. At the beginning of their training, a more senior physician supervises them, and residents are given more responsibility only after they are deemed competent to work alone. They have to read about the effects of fatigue and sleep deprivation. They are provided with more regular supervision from attending physicians.

I envy the schedule of contemporary residents. These changes were phased in after I completed my internship, and I can see their benefits. I remember feeling abandoned in the hospital, trying to figure out how to care for a patient with little assistance. I remember the fatigue of being on call every fourth night for months on end. I remember the errors that occurred while I was exhausted, most modest, but some devastating. I remember feeling distant from my friends, my family, my wife, and our son. I know that in today's system, I would never have been left as the only physician on call for a hospital as vast as Dix on the second night of my residency, or allowed to moonlight on my days off.

But I also wonder how today's trainees will learn all that I learned at Dix. Today's interns and residents have limited opportunities to develop their ability to care for a patient on their own. Instead of admitting a patient who has been seen by no one but an admissions worker assessing vital signs and reviewing demographic data, the residents with whom I now work admit patients only after they have been examined and stabilized by a member of our faculty in the psychiatric Emergency Department. Instead of following a patient throughout his or her first thirty hours of hospitalization, these residents follow the patient for a few hours. Instead of admitting twenty patients and caring for twelve during a day, they admit fewer than ten and care for six.

In this new system, in which residents are constantly passing off patient care to another resident, a different set of errors has arisen. In our hospital, a single patient is handed off four times between residents in a twenty-four-hour period. With each handoff, errors can occur; it's like a game of telephone. And though residents work fewer hours, each of those hours is more full than it was during Osler's era, when patients lingered in the hospital. The hours of today's residents are also filled with new professional responsibilities for transitions in care, responsibilities that pull them away from the bedside.

As a result of these changes, residents are starting to understand their training as a job with clear boundaries: this number of patients for this shift. If a patient with an interesting problem comes in at the end of a shift or if resident is in the middle of working with a patient, he or she still has to leave. Attending physicians often say that they fear this system stunts the growth of the best residents while discouraging weak residents from testing themselves appropriately for the rigors of practice. Attending physicians also worry that residents will learn to practice independently only when they become attending physicians themselves—there are still no duty hour requirements on attending physicians.

In his 1938 commencement speech, Cole advised graduating students, "The hospital should not treat interns as employees, make them punch a time clock (of course figuratively) and provide to the minutest detail the kind and amount of work they shall perform."[9] Less than a century later, we do treat residents as employees, and the time clock is literal. Today's residents log each hour they work with patients as a "duty hour" on online scheduling programs and are penalized if they exceed the allowed hours by mere minutes. In this way, we penalize today's residents for seeing much. Residency training programs are similarly penalized when residents "violate duty hours." Residency training programs that do not obey duty hours and other requirements will receive citations and, if they continue to violate duty hours, lose their accreditation, effectively shuttering a training program for being unprofessional.

So if medical association charters provide the aspirational version of professionalism and pagers enforce professionalism by regulating time, then today's residents are experiencing professionalism as mandated by regulatory agencies. Although the available evidence about the duty hours system suggests that it is improving the didactic education and quality of life of residents, it also suggests that reforming medicine by regulating the hours of physicians is making medicine more costly, fragmented, and bureaucratic.[10]

Reforming medicine through professionalism focuses on the actions of an individual physician; in most such attempts at reform, organizations and committees draft consensus statements describing how an individual physician should behave. As manifestations of such reform measures, pagers have become a way to enforce the requirements of professionalism, to ensure that a physician is available and engaged in his or her responsibilities. The control pagers can exert, however, is limited. In a literal sense, the pagers worked in Libby Zion's case. The nurses paged the intern. The intern replied and remained engaged in her professional responsibilities to her patient. Zion still died in the hospital. And the reform of residency duty hours—the fruit of Zion's death—has endangered Osler's famous model of residency as an opportunity to see much.

The debate about how to preserve Osler's model in the context of duty hours is ongoing, but reformers are increasingly looking beyond pagers and duty hours for other ways to regulate physician behavior.

I am, too. The image I think back to is Osler's vision of the physician as a ship's captain, ferrying his patients across a figurative sea of illness or injury. What if a physician bore responsibility for his or her patients throughout the journey, instead of forever handing off the patient to the next physician? I rarely saw a physician take that kind of responsibility in my residency. Instead, what I saw was a new hope that we could fix medicine not by making physicians more professional or humane but by compelling them to follow the rules of evidence.

During the second year of residency, I began to see patients of my own in the clinic. Unlike call, where I saw them in order of acuity, these patients were scheduled for specific times. Or, to be more accurate, overscheduled, with new patients added throughout the day. To handle the schedule, I learned to be, above all, efficient. Efficiency got me home in time to see our son. Inefficiency kept me in the darkened clinic after everyone else had gone home. During the second year of my residency, Bao challenged my efficiency, persistently dashing my hopes of completing an afternoon clinic before the front desk staff left for the night.

Bao was a forty-three-year-old Vietnamese immigrant who had been adopted at the age of six by a local family. She never really fit in with her adoptive family and eventually exhausted whatever stores of kindness they had. But she had no one else; Bao had never married, never become a mother, never even had a sexual partner. She once told me she felt "as alone as an empty cup."

When the taste of her loneliness grew too bitter, she would come to our Emergency Department. Once a week, twice a week, thrice a week. Chest pain. Suicidal thoughts. Headache. If the Emergency Department physicians and staff could sit with her long enough to fill her cup, she could return home, but the Emergency Department staff usually triaged their time and rarely had sufficient to give to Bao. Eventually, the Emergency Department physicians took to asking, "Bao, on a scale of 1 to 10, which is worse, your chest pain or your thoughts of suicide?" If she answered "chest pain," they paged the on-call internist. If she answered "suicide," it was the on-call psychiatrist's turn to share Bao's lonely cup.

After a couple of rounds of these admissions, the internal medicine and psychiatry services tried to preempt Bao's emergencies. At the beginning of each month, she would have a half-hour appointment with an internal medicine resident. Two weeks later, she would have a half-hour appointment with me, the psychiatry resident. In return, Bao agreed to work with her respective residents instead of visiting the Emergency Department every other night. We fell into a rhythm. Bao began each month with the internist. A few days later, I would read his summary of their encounter in our hospital's electronic medical record. He would assess her somatic complaints, reassure her, and encourage her to discuss her emotions and behaviors with me. When we met, Bao would discuss how she struggled with anxiety and depression. I understood her wavering moods as expressions of her personality structure. She felt empty all the time. Her sense of herself and other people was unstable. The only way to keep people engaged with her was to threaten suicide, and the scars on her arms recorded every failed attempt to keep a friend.

While preparing for one of my monthly meetings, I reviewed the notes from Bao's most recent visit to the internist and saw that she had requested birth control pills. The internist documented that she did not smoke, was not pregnant, and never had cancer, a clotting disorder, liver disease, irregular menstrual bleeds, or a stroke. He concluded that Bao understood the risks and benefits and prescribed Ortho Tri-Cyclen.

Reading the note, I became worried. The internist had asked a series of well-informed questions, but not the most important question.

When Bao arrived, I asked the kind of questions shrinks like. "How's your mood?" "Have you had any unsafe thoughts?" "Any trouble getting to sleep or staying asleep?" Then, I turned to the internist's report.

"I saw that you visited your internist and requested birth control. I was surprised. You always described yourself as a virgin. Has anything changed?"

"I met a man."

"Can you tell me about him?"

85

"My car broke down on the highway. I was on the side of the road, and a police officer helped me call a tow truck. Then he told me he was separated from his wife and he wondered if we could get together sometime. For sex. He told me he liked Asian ladies."

Bao's internist had weighed the available evidence to ensure that the medication he prescribed would not harm her. Oral contraceptives, like any medication, can produce adverse effects. For some people a medication is contraindicated, meaning that they should not take it because the risk of an adverse effect outweighs its potential benefits. A good physician knows and discusses the adverse effects and contraindications of a medication with his or her patients. Bao's internist reviewed the contraindications scrupulously. He did his job.

But he also missed the point of Bao's request. She was preparing for her first sexual encounter after a lifetime of being so ashamed of her body that she frequently harmed herself. An oral contraceptive would, yes, probably prevent her from becoming pregnant, but it would not prevent the cutting that was sure to follow a sexual encounter with a police officer who chose her for her vulnerability and ethnicity.

In medicine, we train physicians to be technicians who gather, assess, and follow evidence. There is much good in doing so. We all want every physician to know the adverse effects and contraindications of a medication before prescribing it to a patient. We all want every physician to know the available evidence for and against a particular test or treatment. In order to be certain that each physician knows and acts upon the best evidence in order to ensure reliable and predictable outcomes, many forces in medicine are compelling physicians to follow evidence-based practices. The problem is that you can follow the best practices and, like Bao's internist, miss what is actually happening in your patient's life.

• • •

When I began medical school, the younger faculty members often drew a distinction between "expert-based" and "evidence-based" medicine. In expert-based medicine, they told us, patients received the care prescribed by an expert, usually a physician, based on his or her clinical experience. In evidence-based medicine, we heard, patients received the care that, after careful consideration of the scientific literature, a physician concluded was best for them. When these faculty members talked, they described evidence-based medicine as a transformative shift from ephemeral opinion to certain evidence.

Many of these faculty members identified themselves as "clinical epidemiologists"—physicians who critically reviewed the available literature using statistical techniques to determine the right course of action for an individual patient. Clinical epidemiology was a relatively new field, pioneered by physicians like David Sackett in the latter half of the twentieth century. Sackett helped transform medicine by first transforming medical education, founding a new medical school at McMaster University in Ontario and doing away with courses or lectures to educate students solely at the bedside and in the library. Instead of listening to their faculty's expert opinions, Sackett's students examined a patient, researched the population-based evidence for the treatment of the patient's condition in the library, and returned to the bedside. Sackett taught generations of McMaster medical students and residents to critically appraise the medical literature so they could use evidence, instead of clinical experience, to determine the best course of treatment for an individual patient.

Gordon Guyatt was one of those McMaster medical students who learned to move between the bedside and the library. When he finished his training, he joined the McMaster faculty as the director of the internal medicine residency and coined a phrase that transmitted the work of his teachers into global medical practice: "evidence-based medicine." From his relatively remote rural outpost in Ontario, Guyatt was setting out to transform medicine.

He found allies among the editorial staff of the *Journal of the American Medical Association* (*JAMA*), one of the world's most influential medical journals. Guyatt popularized the phrase "evidence-based medicine" in a 1992 *JAMA* article. In that article, Guyatt and his colleagues announced evidence-based medicine as "a new paradigm" and a "new philosophy" for medical education and practice. They wrote that, unlike the usual practice of medicine, evidence-based medicine "deals directly with the uncertainties of clinical medicine and has the potential for transforming the education and practice of the next generation of physicians."[1] Guyatt made good on his rhetoric. Over the next eight years, *JAMA* published thirty-two articles by Guyatt and his colleagues, an influential endorsement to evidence-based medicine that spurred its rapid incorporation into medical practice and training. A mere decade after Guyatt introduced the phrase, more than twenty-five hundred peer-reviewed evidence-based medicine papers were being published annually.[2]

The name Guyatt chose was a powerful polemic; who could oppose something that was "evidence-based"? Yet many physicians lamented the rise of evidence-based medicine as "cookbook medicine" that eroded professional autonomy and clinical judgment. In a critical article, two physicians described the declarations in Guyatt's 1992 article "as analogous to a decision to occupy a territory without the involvement of [the] relevant military."[3] Guyatt and other epidemiologists were announcing the reorientation of medicine around their discipline. They did so with few initial contributions from disciplines informed by the humanities and social sciences, disciplines with wisdom about culture, history, and interpersonal relationships. Wisdom, because of its particularity and variability, was pushed to the periphery by evidence-based medicine in favor of efficiency and effectiveness.

The move from expert judgment to evidence-based medicine participates in a larger social trend—what the historian of science Theodore Porter calls the rise of quantification. In *Trust in Numbers: The Pursuit of Objectivity in Science and Public Life*, Porter observed that quantification is the preferred way to communicate about many things, including health and illness, in contemporary life. Physicians speak to patients about prevalence rates, odds of survival, and remission rates. With administrators, we speak about days of uncompensated care, billing variances, and readmission rates. In both cases, numbers win the argument. Porter believed that communicating with numbers was fundamentally distinguished from other forms of communication because it operated as "a technology of distance." Quantification does not depend upon intimate knowledge of a person, or a trusting relationship. Indeed, it discourages them. Knowledge and trust are particular and personal. They are hard to standardize. In order to quantify something, you first have to standardize it, to tame its particular and personal aspects. You have to give up the local in favor of the universal.[4] So when the advocates of evidence-based medicine called for physicians to bring the library to the bedside, they introduced technologies of distance, encouraging physicians to use the numbers, graphs, and formulas that are the strategies of communication particular to quantification. They encouraged physicians to count something rather than to seek understanding of a patient.

Evidence-based medicine proved popular in part because it reached prominence simultaneously with advances in technology, including the availability of journal articles in electronic databases rather than on the dusty shelves of a library, the escalating computing power of statistics programs that automated complex calculations, and the introduction of electronic medical records that enabled the rapid compilation of data. These technologies allowed researchers to answer questions with greater statistical power and precision. Instead of an article written by a senior physician describing favorite methods for, say, reorienting a baby in the breech position during delivery, an article might summarize all the known studies about and quantifying the risks and benefits of the different methods for reorienting a baby. Evidence-based medicine allowed physicians to see health and illness at the population level, which proved to be an alluring vision. Evidence-based medicine provided a state-of-the-art way to see much.

By the time I entered training, evidence-based medicine was synonymous with the future. So in my epidemiology course in my second year of medical school, we learned to critically appraise an article just as Sackett had taught his students to at McMaster, how to read forest plots and funnel plots, and how to interpret chi-squares and p values. The course forced us to think in a new way. Instead of beginning with the patient in front of us, we began with data sets.

Instead of finishing with the uncertain conclusions of the clinical encounter, we ended with precise outcomes. So many of my medical school classmates found this appealing that a third of them took a year off from medical school to earn master's degrees in epidemiology. They threw in their lot with the statistical future of medicine. A few years later, I followed them.

During my psychiatry residency, I was assigned a research mentor who was an expert in schizophrenia. But instead of asking me to gather an Oslerian-style compendium of his expertise, he invited me to co-write a Cochrane review, a statistical, rather than narrative, summary of the effectiveness of a new treatment for schizophrenia.

We were eager to write a Cochrane review because of what it was and what it was not. At the time, many of the clinical trials in medicine were designed, financed, and conducted by pharmaceutical companies. These trials had the power and precision clinical epidemiologists desired—the resulting papers were thick with p values and chi-squares, statistical guarantors of "evidence" as certain as the scriptural citations used by members of a religious community for proof-texting—but they were also riddled with bias. In ways minute and massive, these studies were designed to generate the greatest effects for the manufacturer's drug. So the authors would compare the company's drug to an ineffective dose of another drug, limit the trial to the participants most likely to benefit from the treatment, or pay academic leaders to run favorable trials. When one looked closely at these papers, they looked less like scientific reports and more like marketing pamphlets.

And, indeed, they often became marketing pamphlets. Although the papers were published in medical journals, their most telling presentations came at lunches and dinners sponsored by Big Pharma. Pharmaceutical representatives would reprint favorable studies on glossy paper and hand them to physicians along with a roast beef sandwich in a hospital conference room. Or a leading physician would introduce the study in a projected presentation while local physicians ate overpriced meals in the backroom of a steakhouse.

My research mentor eschewed these kinds of studies and the corrupting influence Big Pharma has on medicine. He favored the clean lines of clinical epidemiology, and the cleanest lines in all of clinical epidemiology are those drawn by a Cochrane review. Every medical school and residency lecture by a clinical epidemiologist included a picture of a pyramid. The bottom of the pyramid was a wide base labeled "expert opinion," a visual rejoinder to experts that their expertise and opinion were neither exceptional nor refined. A hierarchy developed along the ascending steps of the pyramid: case reports to case series, cohort studies, clinical trials, critical appraisals of the literature, systematic reviews, meta-analyses, and, at the apex, Cochrane reviews. With each step, the quality of the evidence was said to increase.

In one way, the pyramid undid Osler, whose life's work was focused on the base—expert opinion, case reports, and case series—in favor of clinical epidemiologists with the statistical knowledge to conduct systematic reviews and meta-analyses. You could be an excellent clinical epidemiologist without having any skill in conducting either a physical examination or an autopsy. If Osler described medical training and practice as a conversation between the bedside and the morgue, Cochrane reviews present them as a conversation between the bedside and the database. In another way, the pyramid was simply an updated version of Osler's proposal. At each new level of the pyramid, the designated study included ever more patients until, from the apex, the Cochrane review, a physician could see the health not just of individual patients but of whole populations. Seeing much was still the goal.

• • •

Cochrane reviews are named after their inspiration, Archibald "Archie" Leman Cochrane, a pioneering British physician and epidemiologist who was present at many of the seminal moments of twentieth-century European history. Born into a wealthy Scottish tweed-making family whose patriarch was killed at the Battle of Gaza, Archie received psychoanalysis with disciples of Freud in Berlin and Vienna, served in an ambulance unit in the Spanish Civil War, earned a medical degree, and enlisted in the Royal Army Medical Corps as a medical officer. The Germans took him prisoner during his first military action and, because he had learned German during his course of psychoanalysis, put him in charge of providing medical care for twenty thousand fellow prisoners in the Dulag, a POW transit camp. Cochrane never had a traditional medical practice; from the start of his career, he was asked to manage the health of a population. In the camps, he was struck by how little evidence was available to guide him in selecting for or against a particular intervention. In what would become his habit, Cochrane ran simple clinical trials in which he would divide his patients into separate treatment groups to determine which treatment was most effective. When he was released from the POW camp, Cochrane returned to London to continue his medical training. He studied there with Austin Bradford Hill, a British epidemiologist famed both for identifying the association between cigarette smoking and lung cancer and for conducting the first randomized controlled trial.[5] In a randomized controlled trial, participants are randomly assigned to different interventions, a design that reduces the influence of biases or prejudice toward or against a particular intervention. In Hill's randomized controlled trials, Cochrane believed he had found a way to fix medicine.

The problem facing medicine, Cochrane later wrote, was fundamentally a question of determining which interventions worked and how these interventions should be distributed among a population. Even as a POW physician, he had been surprised at how little his own interventions altered the health of his patients:

> Under the best conditions one would have expected an appreciable mortality; there in the Dulag I expected hundreds to die of diphtheria alone in the absence of specific therapy. In point of fact there were only four deaths, of which three were due to gunshot wounds inflicted by the Germans. This excellent result had, of course, nothing to do with the therapy they received or my clinical skill. It demonstrated, on the other hand, very clearly the relative unimportance of therapy

in comparison with the recuperative power of the human body. On one occasion, when I was the only doctor there, I asked the German Stabsarzt for more doctors to help me cope with these fantastic problems. He replied, "Nein! Ärzte sind überflüssig." ("No! Doctors are superfluous.") I was furious and even wrote a poem about it; later I wondered if he was wise or cruel; he was certainly right."[6]

From this experience, Cochrane learned to distrust received wisdom, medical dogma, and the necessity of medical treatment.

Cochrane knew, though, that there were times when having access to a physician was essential to health. At those times, he was deeply committed to equality in healthcare. So when the British government founded the National Health Service in 1948 to provide and finance healthcare through tax payments, Cochrane was a strong supporter. In time, though, he feared that its free services were leading patients to seek, and physicians to provide, all the possible treatments available. The solution, Cochrane believed, was for epidemiologists to inform physicians and the National Health Service about which of the possible interventions should be applied to a particular patient—he made the utilitarian argument that healthcare systems should provide only the interventions with the most favorable costs and risk-benefit profiles, the interventions demonstrated to be efficient and effective. In 1971 he delivered a series of lectures on the role randomized controlled trials could play in the National Health Service. Published as the book *Effectiveness and Efficiency: Random Reflections on Health Services*, the lectures became a cornerstone of clinical epidemiology and evidence-based medicine.

Cochrane's ideas influenced not only David Sackett and his students at McMaster as they developed evidence-based medicine, but also the British health-services researcher Iain Chalmers. In his book, Cochrane had called for an international registry of randomized trials. Later he called specifically for a "critical summary, by specialty or subspecialty, adapted periodically, of all relevant randomised controlled trials."[7] Chalmers responded to Cochrane's challenge by collecting all the randomized controlled trials he could find for his own field of study and organizing them into the Oxford Database of Perinatal Trials, an electronic resource for physicians and policy makers.

Chalmers's work addressed several problems with randomized controlled trials. One trouble with such trials is that their results apply only to the participants of the particular study, not necessarily to the population to which a physician might want to apply them. Another is that two well-conducted randomized control trials may reach contradictory conclusions. Chalmers's solution was to synthesize the findings into a single review, called a systematic review.

Systematic reviews are both collections, in which are gathered all the high-quality studies on a particular topic, and syntheses, integrated findings aimed at answering a particular question. In 1989, Chalmers and his colleagues published *A Guide to Effective Care in Pregnancy and Childbirth*, a two-volume collection of systematic reviews that collectively proved that many common interventions in obstetrics were not only unhelpful but also dangerous.[8] Chalmers dreamed of writing similar reviews for the entirety of medicine, and in 1992 the research and development division of the National Health Service helped him toward that goal by creating a center to conduct and publish similar systematic reviews; they appointed Chalmers as the first director and named the organization after his inspiration, Archie Cochrane.

Today, the Cochrane Collaboration is an international nonprofit organization staffed by 30,000 volunteer patients, practitioners, and researchers in 120 countries. Together, the members have written 6,000 reviews of specific interventions in medicine. Cochrane reviews are like Wikipedia with better math; the work is crowd-sourced, with reviews edited and updated regularly, but the resulting knowledge is appraised and synthesized using biostatistics. They are available worldwide, and are free for practitioners and policy makers in low- and middle-income countries. The reviews are self-consciously characterized as the best evidence in contemporary medicine.[9]

In a sly way, I think they are also a testament to Cochrane's suspicion that physicians are superfluous to healthcare.

My mentor and I were assigned to write a Cochrane review of a drug to treat schizophrenia, the chronic, often disabling, psychotic disorder. The drug, paliperidone, was new but familiar; it is a metabolite of risperidone, a widely prescribed drug that chiefly works by blocking dopamine receptors in the brain. When risperidone's patent ran out, the manufacturer's profits withered, and they introduced paliperidone to take its place. Paliperidone had a few novel characteristics—a long-acting version has some practical advantages over risperidone's long-acting version—and we were eager to evaluate it.

I managed to do the work during the margins of the day, in the clinic when a patient cancelled or from home while our son was sleeping. The review required no funding or regulatory approval, only my time and a laptop capable of running the Cochrane Collaboration's proprietary software.

Writing the review felt like building a ready-made. Using the Collaboration I searched the international medical literature, from which I got thousands of pages of journal articles, presentation abstracts, and regulatory filings. My mentor and I read through them, identified additional references, and drew up a list of all the possible studies. Then we graded each of the studies based on criteria provided to us by Cochrane headquarters. If the study was the kind of randomized controlled trial that Archie liked, we included it; if not, we excluded it. A lot of this work seemed like something robots will eventually do, but we kept on, abstracting data from each of the included studies, entering it into a Cochrane-provided program, and watching as the program returned a statistical summary. We interpreted the stats, wrote a narrative summary, edited it based upon peer review, and then sent our evidence-based, state-of-the-art systematic review off into the world.

It stood little chance against the marketing pamphlets. Their conclusions were extravagant; ours were measured. They offered physicians glossy, full-color ads with pictures of disheveled men and women on one side and—thanks to the miracle of paliperidone!—

clean and confident ones on the other; we issued a several-hundred-page, single-spaced document whose only pictures were forest plots and data tables. Though we found little evidence that paliperidone was superior to its less expensive parent compound, the manufacturer grossed billions of dollars on it. Despite following the best practices and selecting and synthesizing the best possible evidence, I felt as though the experience had been both inefficient and ineffective. The review's selection criteria limited our analysis to the randomized controlled trials of paliperidone, but the only people conducting randomized controlled trials of paliperidone were researchers funded by the manufacturer, so our review was a carefully conducted analysis of all the marketing pamphlet studies it was meant to displace. In a funny way, our review unintentionally extended the evidence-based imprimatur to paliperidone.

And the studies with which we worked rarely answered the questions practitioners need to answer when considering whether to use paliperidone for a particular patient. Those studies excluded people with unstable social circumstances or substance-abuse problems and those who historically did not respond to risperidone. Of course, many psychiatric patients fit all three of these criteria. Worse, most of those studies lasted only six weeks—six weeks for a condition we believe is chronic. So if a patient asks me about the long-term effects of a medication I am supposed to recommend that he or she take for the rest of his or her life, the evidence-based answer remains little more than a shrug of the shoulders.

• • •

Randomized trials are designed for the kingdom of quantification, a place where we can readily measure standardized outcomes. They are hard to relate to the world of patients like Bao. Bao's very self was porous, profoundly dependent upon how others—whether an internist, a police officer, or a psychiatrist—related to her. Counting anything connected with her first required imposing a decision about where she began and where she ended.

During my writing of the Cochrane review—it took two years of nights and weekends—I was seeing a lot of Bao. She had had sex with the police officer, and while she had not gotten pregnant, she became suicidal again when he stopped returning her calls. In the months that followed, she frequently returned to the Emergency Department, now always with thoughts or gestures of suicide. No need to call the internist. Instead, I would be paged away from other patients once a week so that I could evaluate her.

I would pull up a chair and ask her what was going on. She would roll up her sleeves to show bright red lines on her forearm or dig into her purse and wordlessly present me with an empty pill bottle like a defiant child. I would measure the depth of the cuts or count the number of pills she had swallowed, and if I thought my calculations indicated a gesture, a bid for attention, I would send her home. If they added up to a serious attempt, a threat on her life, I would admit her upstairs. I had no Cochrane review or evidence-based tool to guide my decision whether to discharge or admit Bao, but I tried to quantify the problem anyway because I had too little clinical judgment. I was trying to see her as a medical problem to be summed and solved: When Bao first walked into her internist's office requesting an oral contraceptive, her problem was that she had a history of emotional instability and interpersonal conflict that suggested she was headed for an unhealthy sexual encounter.

Or: Bao's problem was that a law enforcement officer had violated his code of conduct and propositioned Bao because of her ethnicity and vulnerability.

Or: Bao's problem was that, as Archie Cochrane might have said, physicians were involved in a decision they should not have been.

But in a hospital run according to the logic of evidence-based medicine, Bao's problem was simply that she wanted to have sex without getting pregnant. So her internist asked questions about the adverse effects that evidence-based reviews have most consistently associated with oral contraceptives.

These kinds of decisions are made daily in the clinic and hospital. A patient presents with a problem, and a physician offers a medical interpretation of the problem. The physician-as-technician then efficiently and effectively selects an evidence-based intervention for the problem, having first made the assumption that the patient needs a medical intervention. Evidence-based medicine guides like Cochrane reviews will never be able to rate how suitable a particular sexual partner might be or whether a patient will become suicidal after having sex with a police officer. Archie Cochrane had asked whether physicians should intervene, an apt question for practitioners in the National Health Service, where all services were funded and provided by the British government. In the National Health Service, a physician who saw Bao and elected to prescribe neither an oral contraceptive nor a course of psychotherapy would still be paid. When the Cochrane Collaboration was created, however, it advanced Archie Cochrane's ideas into countries with very different financing systems. In these systems, practitioners are paid only if they do something or help someone achieve a measurable outcome. In these systems, a practitioner receives little payment if he or she does not prescribe an intervention of some kind for a patient like Bao. In this different context, Cochrane reviews do not ask if doctors should perform a medical intervention; they ask which medical intervention doctors should perform. The authors of Cochrane reviews know (and repeatedly state) the limits of the knowledge they generate, but those limits are forgotten when we turn that knowledge into scripts for clinical encounters where an intervention is presumed. In a clinic, a doctor must efficiently and effectively intervene in the life of a patient like Bao, even when Archie Cochrane himself might have said "No! Doctors are superfluous." In medicine, we rarely recall Cochrane's warning. Instead, we are working to bring his style of epidemiological findings into clinical practice, to bring the bedside ever closer to the dataset, and to introduce ever more technologies of distance between physicians and patients.

seven

CHECKLISTS AND DANCE LESSONS

A shrill tune came from the consult pager on my belt. I slipped the pager from its holster and read the text message: "STAT consult. Pt uncontrollable. Aliens attacking." Not wanting attacking aliens to gain control of the hospital, the city, or our proud planet, I holstered the pager, collected my medical student, and headed for the stairs and the uncontrollable patient.

The cardiac catheterization laboratory was on the other side of the medical center, so we walked quickly through the skyways and stairwells that connected one hospital tower to the next. I was a fourth-year resident on the consult service, available to physicians throughout the medical center when a patient had an urgent psychiatric concern. Calling a consult, as it is called, often feels like asking for reinforcements. You call a consult because you feel pinned down by your responsibilities. Many of my psychiatric consults were mundane—a surgeon did not know what to say to a despondent father, an internist wanted to know why a homeless woman was declining the expensive treatment he recommended—but others were momentous. I met with burn ward patients who were sneaking off the unit to smoke crack and obstetric patients doubled over with birth pains from delusional pregnancies. From the staccato text message on the pager, this consult sounded like it might be memorable.

When we arrived in the catheter lab, a nurse was holding the door open. "You with psych?" I nodded. "She's all yours. Cuckoo-catchoo."

Fifteen yards away, a woman was standing alone in the center of the room. Her head was tilted up, her eyes looking into the overhead surgical spotlight. She held her arms slightly out from her sides, taut as a pulled cord, so that even as she stood still, she appeared to be moving. She looked like a rocket pointing toward a horizon beyond the ceiling.

Ten yards away from her, the cardiology fellow stood with his arms crossed over the cath lab's now-scuttled morning schedule. He turned, looked at me, and shook his head, as if to say, "See what happens when we take one of your patients?" He had the patient's medical record pulled up on a screen, and I scanned it quickly. Public insurance. Distant address. Name, Aruna. Age, sixty-six. Admitted last night for a heart attack. No history of mental illness. A terse history and physical completed by an on-call intern. A few lines of abbreviations and acronyms signed by the cardiology fellow. Two EKGs. One pre-op cardiac catheterization checklist with a flurry of checkmarks.

Five yards away from her, a security officer stood in his interview stance, his hands resting above his gun, his body bladed forty-five degrees toward Aruna. We knew each other from around the hospital. He nodded in Aruna's direction and put out his hands, silently asking me if he should put hands on her. I waved him off and stood opposite him, facing Aruna obliquely. She looked calm but determined.

"Aruna?"

"Not my name."

"What should I call you?"

"Shhh. Not telling."

"Where are you from?"

"Not here."

"Me neither. Where are you from?"

"Up there! Headed home."

Aruna was determinedly alone in the middle of that thousand-bed hospital, growing city, doomed planet. She was waiting to leave us all behind, so my first task was to interest her in those of us still tethered to the ground.

• • •

Visiting a contemporary hospital can feel a lot like being in an airport: the building is secured, the delays are unexplained, and you take your clothes off in front of strangers to prevent attacks from distant threats. Working in a contemporary hospital can also feel a lot like being employed at an airport: as medical practitioners, our time is regulated, our speech is scripted, and our interactions are impersonal. What surprises many patients and physicians is that these correspondences are intentional.

We talk all the time about coordinating care in contemporary medicine. In today's clinics and hospitals, the care of patients is constantly being handed off among physicians, nurses, pharmacists, and other practitioners. So when we talk about coordinating care, we do not mean that these various practitioners should match their disparate plans with the desires of the patients. What we mean is that the cards—cardiology—nurse and the cards fellow and the psych consultant should work together the way engineers do: each of us works on a different part of the same patient, so we need to work in sequence to provide the complex procedures and services that constitute contemporary healthcare. The celebrated way that we do so is with processes adopted from industrial engineering, processes like the checklist in Aruna's record.

Which leads us back to the airport. Checklists were first used by airlines as way to standardize the actions of a pilot to increase safety. Before entering the plane, the pilot would verify, say, that the wheel chocks were in place and the trim tabs were neutral. A good pilot would always have checked those things on his or her own. But even the best and the most experienced sometimes forget to check. Accidents occur when people forget, and the failure to use checklists, or the misuse of checklists, has been identified as a cause of many an airplane crash. Now, before they start engines, take off, or land a plane, a pilot and his or her crew complete a checklist, constantly reconfiguring the plane to match the checklist. The airline checklists draw on decades of evidence to protect the lives of passengers.[1]

The checklist in Aruna's chart represented a similar attempt to operationalize the findings generated by epidemiologists over the previous half-century. Those findings were buried in thousands of articles, and, even when systematically summarized in something like a Cochrane review, the documents ran for dozens of pages. It is impossible to use such hefty tomes to coordinate the care of an efficient cardiac cath lab. A catheterization team has no more than twenty or thirty minutes to push a thin tube against the blood's vital current and move upstream from an artery in the arm or groin or neck until it reaches the plaque in the artery that is damming up the current. Many things can go wrong—the serious issues include bleeding and infection—but a cath lab team can prevent most of them by following the known rules for the procedure. So as each patient waited to enter the lab, a nurse was responsible for filling out a checklist, based on a series of evidence-based reviews of the factors associated with adverse outcomes during cardiac catheterization. The nurse would ask if the patient had a history of bleeding or had recently taken any of a number of medications that increased his or her risk of bleeding. The cath lab team would not perform the procedure until the checklist was completed.[2]

Over the past decade, an obsession for checklists gripped medicine. We developed checklists for preoperative clearances and intraoperative procedures but also to assess symptoms of depression, to reconcile discharge medications, and to standardize everything we can.

The leading public advocate for the use of checklists in medicine has been the surgeon-writer Atul Gawande. In his academic career, he has piloted checklists for surgical procedures that have been endorsed by the World Health Organization and subsequently implemented in hospitals throughout the world. He also wrote a best seller, *The Checklist Manifesto*, about how checklists protect people from both anticipated and unanticipated problems when they are engaged in complex technical tasks that require coordinated efforts, tasks like flying a plane or catheterizing the vessels of a sixty-six-year-old's heart.[3]

The checklist had been completed for Aruna, an elderly Thai immigrant. She spoke little English, so her daughter-in-law had provided most of the information. The nurse had verified Aruna's name, the procedure, her cardiac history, her medications, and more. Check, check, check.

And yet the procedure failed in ways that the checklist could not have anticipated. Checklists excel at preventing the common errors associated with cardiac catheterization in the medical literature. In the peer-reviewed literature on cardiac catheterization, there are tens of thousands of published articles. The checklist was a single page that rendered this knowledge useful in the quick-moving cockpit of a contemporary cath lab.

The nurse had ten patients in the holding bay waiting their turn in one of the hospital's procedural rooms. So as the nurse was making her rounds, she used the checklist to review Aruna's allergies, medications, informed consent, healthcare proxy, and more, then signed off, clearing Aruna for takeoff from the preoperative suite. The checklist was necessary, but it was insufficient for Aruna's case because it assessed only the potential for adverse effects associated with the scheduled procedure, not Aruna herself.

Mumbling was not on the nurse's checklist, but Aruna's mumbling was the first sign that she was not ready for catheterization.

When I arrived, the family—daughter-in-law, son, and three grandchildren—was still in the waiting room. I joined them in the hallway, introducing myself and asking for a little more background on Aruna. They told me she had spent her life in a small town in southern Thailand. She had seven children, six of whom still lived in Thailand. Aruna visited her oldest son in America annually, but she had always returned home until two months earlier, when her husband had died and she had moved in with her son's family.

Aruna minded her grandkids when their parents were out, cooked most of the meals, and occasionally visited fellow Thai immigrants in the area. Her family insisted she had no history of strange behavior or unusual thoughts. She talked about wanting to return to Thailand, where her other children still lived, but never about returning to an extraterrestrial home.

I asked whether she was on any medications. Aruna's daughter-in-law said no. I asked about drugs or alcohol. Aruna's son shook his head. My med student asked the family whether she took any herbal medicines or supplements. Aruna's daughter-in-law nodded.

Aruna had felt constipated and fatigued lately, so a Thai acquaintance had given her kratom to alleviate her symptoms on the day before she was hospitalized. Kratom is a Thai herbal remedy that, like many drugs, works differently at different doses. At low doses, kratom is a stimulant, but at high doses, it is an analgesic; at low doses, it acts like cocaine, at high doses like opium.[4] Aruna had her heart attack while using low doses but had continued to chew a supply of kratom in the hospital. While the nurse was completing the checklist, Aruna was mumbling because she was chewing enough kratom to experience its opiate-like effects. As she waited, she had become delusional and euphoric.

With time, rest, and some water, Aruna improved, but the catheterization had to wait. Her checklist cleared her for the procedure, but her intoxication meant that the procedure was delayed until Aruna returned to earth.

• • •

A patient high on kratom is rare in contemporary clinics and hospitals, but inconsistent results from checklists are all too frequent. Often we complete our checklists but patients like Aruna still experience a bad outcome. Aruna did not have any of the bad outcomes the checklists were intended to prevent. She did not bleed out or develop an infection during her morning in the cath lab. But as checklists encourage physicians, nurses, and other practitioners to focus on common errors, they draw attention away from uncommon errors. Aruna was the victim of an uncommon error that was missed by the checklist. Checklist writers are aware of this reality and accept that in catching common errors they might miss some uncommon ones. Checklists are a utilitarian tool, designed to maximize benefit and minimize risk. To be useful, checklists have to be brief and can never include everything that might go wrong. These are accepted features of checklists.

Checklists offer distillations of evidence-based medicine into algorithms and scripts that improve quality and safety. And they can aid moral reasoning. But when a practitioner bases the entire encounter with a patient on checklists, they become obstacles to moral reasoning. Checklists also work better in some settings than in others because different settings rely more or less on people working together. Neither of these issues is an accepted feature of checklists, and neither is what those in the quality and safety movement have in mind when advocating for their use.

For the past twenty years, advocates in the quality and safety movement have argued that the problem with healthcare is that medicine does not consistently and safely deliver the best treatments.[5] Their proposed solution is to transform the delivery of medical care using efficacious processes pioneered in high-risk industries like aviation. Medicine, like aviation, involves dangerous tasks that require coordinated efforts. Quality-improvement advocates like to quote a favorite analogy, first offered by the pediatrician Lucian Leape in 1994: the number of people who die because of errors in American hospitals each day is equivalent to the deaths from the crash of a full jumbo jet.[6] The analogy had the startling force Leape desired. If a jumbo jet crashed every day, people would be outraged at the airline industry, and Leape's analogy launched a cycle of public outrage—op-eds, Sunday night news shows, congressional hearings, and government funding—at the deadly errors occurring in medicine. Two decades later, leaders at every level of medicine agree that quality and safety need to be improved in hospitals and clinics, and the jumbo jet story is repeated like an origin myth for the reform of medicine through quality improvement. The rhetorical appeal of Leape's logic has won broad support.

Regulators have certainly embraced this logic. Over the past twenty years, a growing group of regulators have promoted quality improvement techniques as the way to improve patient safety.[7] Resident physicians are now required to conduct quality-improvement projects in order to complete their training.[8] Governmental regulators and insurers assess hospitals on the basis of their performance on standardized quality-improvement measures, rewarding high performers and penalizing low performers. Legislators have enshrined quality improvement in healthcare reform measures.

The intentions are good—to eliminate common mistakes by adopting quality and safety measures such as checklists—but the efforts have inconsistently translated into improvements. Despite two decades of growing attention to quality and safety, the most recent estimates are that the equivalent of two to five jumbo-jet-loads of patients now die each day in American hospitals from preventable errors.[9]

The leaders of the quality movement are aware of this and concerned. Mark Chassin, the president and CEO of the Joint Commission, the leading regulator of American hospitals, recently wrote that even though "hospitals have devoted considerable time, energy, and resources to solving safety and quality problems . . . improvements have been slow and have not spread."[10] Chassin expressed frustration that quality and safety measures have failed in hospitals worldwide, even though similar measures have led to remarkable successes in other industrial sites that, like hospitals, have large staffs tasked with dangerous activities. While Chassin and other quality-improvement leaders lament the results, they insist that the solution remains the adoption of quality and safety techniques pioneered by engineers in industries like aviation. They have a point: two to five jumbo jets do not crash daily.

Industrial engineers have greatly increased the quality and safety of industrial processes in many industries in part by employing the quality-improvement principles developed by W. Edwards Deming, an American mathematician who helped revive Japan following World War II. During the reconstruction of postwar Japan, Deming became familiar with a generation of Japanese leaders through his work conducting a census for the U.S. Army. Then, in a series of lectures, he taught thousands of Japanese engineers how to use statistical methods to improve industrial processes by controlling variations in performance. These lectures became the basis for Deming's later career as a business school professor and author; he summarized his lessons in bulleted messages: Fourteen Points for the Transformation of Management, a four-part System of Profound Knowledge, a list of eight Lesser Categories of Obstacles, and the Seven Deadly Diseases of Management.[11]

Deming's students and intellectual heirs have applied his principles to many different industries, and some, like Lucian Leape, have applied them to the practice of medicine in an attempt to reduce adverse outcomes and improve the efficiency of healthcare. The trouble is that, as near as I can tell, Deming himself never worked in healthcare or applied his principles to healthcare, and healthcare has important differences from the other industries in which he did work.

Still, I share the frustration of quality-improvement leaders with our ongoing failure to protect the lives of our patients. At Denver Health, I work as a physician quality officer, responsible for identifying errors small and large, reporting them to the relevant agencies, and developing processes to prevent the recurrence of these errors. We ought to prevent these errors, and what I admire about the quality improvement movement is that it is attempting to prevent not just some but *all* preventable errors.

What I question is the assumption that principles designed for industries like aviation will work best in medicine. The safety record of airplane travel is admirable, but I appreciate little else about the experience. When I fly, the pilot speaks to me, not with me, through an overhead speaker. I usually feel less like a person and more like cargo along for the ride. If we continue to apply this kind of quality improvement to hospitals and clinics, will the interactions between physicians and other practitioners with patients become as anonymous and pragmatic as the relationship I have with pilots? Will physicians, nurses, and other practitioners believe that we have done our job as long as we complete our checklists even if, as with Aruna, we miss what is going on with the patient?

I hope there is something about medicine that makes being a healthcare practitioner different from flying an airplane. In pursuit of that difference, we have to look beyond industrial engineering and its checklists. We need dance lessons.

• • •

Though Deming never worked in medicine, Ludwig Wittgenstein, another twentieth-century intellectual who studied engineering, did. Wittgenstein was, by many accounts, the most original philosopher of the twentieth century, but when World War II broke out, he resigned his post as a philosophy professor at the University of Cambridge to work as a porter in a London hospital. While Cochrane spent the war doctoring a prison-camp population and Deming spent it expanding industrial processes, Wittgenstein spent it caring directly for the ill. He transported patients, dressed wounds, and prepared ointments.[12]

I am fascinated by his decision to shift as a student from engineer to philosopher and then, as a professor, to shift from philosopher to porter. I have spent my adult life climbing the lower rungs of the medical ladder and find Wittgenstein's voluntary descent baffling. Who gives up an endowed chair to ferry patients around the hospital?

It was the checklist in Aruna's chart that started me thinking about Wittgenstein the porter. Wittgenstein had an aphorism—"Obeying a rule is a practice"—that reminded me a bit of the checklists. After all, what is a checklist but a kind of rule? But what does the aphorism mean? Does Wittgenstein mean you have to practice rule following? If so, which rules? Whose rules? Wittgenstein's aphorism is dense, a bit of gnomic wisdom folded in upon itself, seemingly nothing like the declarative instructions on a checklist. Thinking about it, I went searching for my old copy of the philosopher Charles Taylor's essay "To Follow a Rule," in which he explored Wittgenstein's aphorism.[13]

In the essay, Taylor observed that for two or more people to follow a rule, they need to share certain understandings that cannot be stated in the rule itself. These shared and assumed understandings, Taylor showed, are the social practices that make the rule possible. Yet Taylor observed that today we tend to focus on the rules rather than the social practices upon which they depend. We imagine a person following the rule without considering how the person relates to other people or to his or her own body. To understand Wittgenstein's aphorism, Taylor argued, we have to fully consider these relationships and how they affect our ability to follow rules.

Taylor's essay clarified for me one problem with how we are attempting to use checklists in hospitals today. When we apply rules developed by one group of people to a second group of people, we do not adequately consider the different social practices of the first and second groups. We focus on the outcomes resulting from applying the rules in different communities, but we neglect the context in which we apply the rules. So one problem with checklists is that they are developed in one social context and exported to other, different contexts. A checklist that works in Milan may not work in Muleshoe.

By this logic, it is less surprising that checklists are not transforming medicine in the hoped-for way. For a checklist to be a successful social practice in healthcare, it must account for many different relationships: that between the physician or other practitioner and other employees of the hospital or clinic, that between the physician and patient, that between the physician or practitioner and his or her own body, and that between a patient and his or her own body. Physicians and patients are abstractions, but when people participate in these social roles, they are embodied in particular bodies and particular social roles. What my reading of Taylor made clear to me is that medicine is a social practice. To renew medicine, we need to learn less from industrial engineering processes, whose goal is to produce the same outcome each time, and more from other social practices.

In his essay, Taylor offered dancing as a paradigmatic social practice because it involves a constant interplay between people, a give-and-take. We could likewise see offering and receiving medical care as a social practice akin to dancing. Viewed this way, medicine requires a common rhythm between physician and patient. Each has a body—an illness can exist only within the body of a patient—and each stands in relationship to the other: a physician needs an ill person to care for. Taylor wrote, "A very important feature of human action is rhythming, cadence. Every apt, coordinated gesture has a certain flow. When you lose this, as occasionally happens, you fall into confusion, your actions become inept and uncoordinated."[14]

Following Taylor, one way to account for my meeting with Aruna in the cath lab is that we were engaged in a kind of dance. She was deciding whether she could trust me, and I was trying to keep up with her—not with her mind or her racing thoughts, but with Aruna in her body. You cannot dance with an idea, only with a partner in relationship with yourself, and to dance together you have to develop a common rhythm.

At the same time, comparing dancing to medicine may seem difficult because two dancers are perceived as equals in the relationship, whereas a physician and patient are perceived as engaged in an imbalanced relationship controlled by the physician. That day in the cath lab, Aruna was an immigrant grandmother in the strange world of the hospital. Each of us present in the room stood in a different relationship to her. The nurse was thinking about how to quickly and safely prepare Aruna and nine other patients for the procedure. The cards fellow was thinking about the arteries of her heart. The security officer was thinking about whether Aruna posed a danger and needed to be restrained. I was thinking about how to calm her so the cath lab personnel could go about their business and I could head to the next consult. And all of us were foreign to Aruna. Perhaps it should come as little surprise that she received the whole situation as alien and desired to rocket away.

Years later, I wonder how Aruna's care would have differed if someone had explained the steps of the procedure, as a lead dancer might explain them to his or her dance partner when they were learning a new dance. I wonder whether telling Aruna, or her daughter-in-law, why we were asking the questions on the checklist could have stopped her from chewing the kratom and launching on her psychotic journey.

• • •

Engineers design, implement, and correct a process. They judge its success by how efficiently and effectively it produces a desired outcome. Using the checklist with Aruna in the cath lab produced the desired outcome—she neither bled out nor developed an infection—but the checklist clearly missed what was going on with Aruna. She was actively chewing kratom while the nurse completed it. Aruna and the nurse were physically close to each other but remained strangers, and maybe the problem with the checklist was that it was too much like a written rule for an engineering process and not enough like a dance lesson.

We often conceive of medicine as controlling the body, which is why analogies to industrial engineering, where a worker is responsible for the inanimate object he or she manipulates, carry such currency in contemporary medicine. We compare physicians to airplane pilots, implicitly likening our bodies to airplanes, machines controlled by physicians. An airplane pilot is responsible for flying a plane, but patients and practitioners have a mutual responsibility to care for a body. When we remember that medicine is a human activity like dancing, we can account for the mutual responsibility of both dancers.

We could also remember that just as a dancer may lead at one moment and be led at another, our roles as patients and physicians are fluid: all of us who are physicians at present will some day be patients ourselves and will have to learn those unfamiliar steps. Remembering the way our roles change over time—from patient to physician to patient—is part of understanding medicine as a social practice with common rhythms. We learn medicine through participation in relationships that are like dances—formed by apprenticing to expert physicians and listening to patients—with rules learned through social practices.

In psychiatry, the technical name for the relationship, or dance, between a physician and a patient is the therapeutic alliance, the shared commitment between physician and patient to seek the well-being of a patient. Even though we have ample evidence that developing therapeutic alliances improves health outcomes, quality and safety measures such as checklists are rarely used to assess therapeutic alliances.[15] Quality and safety measures improve easily quantifiable outcomes but are poorly designed for assessing and encouraging the social practices through which outcomes improve.

To borrow Taylor's words, one way to explain the problems of contemporary medicine is to say that we have lost the shared rhythms and coordinated flow of the physician-patient relationship; we have become "inept and uncoordinated." If we formulate the problem of medicine this way, the solution would not be more rules like checklists, but something akin to dance lessons—practices that would rehabituate physicians and patients to the rhythms of a therapeutic alliance. Perhaps if we want to obey our well-intentioned rules for patient safety and quality, we first need to look closer at practices like the therapeutic alliance. In establishing a positive relationship between physician and patient, the rules could begin to seem more like fluid steps of a dance than the measured steps of an engineering process. For Aruna, it would have meant developing enough of a relationship with her before wheeling her into the cath lab that she would have disclosed her use of kratom.

• • •

Around the same time I was learning from Aruna, the most esteemed teacher in Chapel Hill finished teaching a similar lesson. Dean Smith, the legendary coach of the University of North Carolina basketball team for more than three decades, was beloved around town for helping to integrate its restaurants and its athletic conference, for setting aside the sponsorship money he received from shoe companies to help his players, and for insisting that his basketball players be students. His players remembered him as the best teacher they ever had. They said that even though he retired as the winningest coach in college basketball history, he never talked about winning. Instead of discussing the outcome of a game, he described its process, telling his players, "Play hard. Play smart. Play together."[16] In fact, his players remember that the only time they heard him talk about winning was after an unexpected defeat in the national championship semifinals. He retired soon afterward and never coached again. When I heard the story from his players, I wondered whether it meant that Dean Smith retired when coaching became less about process and more about outcomes. I never had a chance to ask him. By the time I arrived in Chapel Hill, he was often mentioned around campus, but rarely seen.

And the university's medical center, like medical centers across the world, was shifting from processes to outcomes. To fix our clinics and hospitals, we were told to run them like factories. To fix healthcare, we were told to perfect our checklists and scripts. No one mentioned dance lessons, or therapeutic alliances, or an old coach's emphasis on process over outcomes.

"You see what is going on in this picture? It's a battleship in the middle of the ocean, moving along at cruising speed. Alongside it is an oil tanker. You see those tubes there? What do you think they're doing? That's right, the tanker is refilling the battleship in the middle of the ocean. You realize how difficult that is? Massive ships, moving fast, in the middle of the ocean. Thousands of gallons of fuel. A lot could go wrong. You know how many times they have crashed? Never. Never! How do they do it? Both ships are staffed with hundreds of young people, fresh out of high school. They are neither experienced nor skilled, but the ships have never crashed, because they follow a well-designed process."

The basement speaker clicks to the next slide. "What about this? It's a restaurant. Hundreds of meals every night. Each meal made from scratch. Each meal modified for the diner. You don't like cilantro? They leave it out of the pad thai. Gluten-free? They make your salad without croutons. I like cilantro and croutons myself, but more than anything, I like my meal the way I want it, and this place does it, night in and night out. They have twenty chefs in this kitchen. None of these guys is famous, but they make hundreds of perfect meals every night. How do they do it? See those computers above their kitchen stations? They are following standard work."

The speaker gestures to his assistant to pass out a packet of articles. As she circulates around the room, he continues. "Over the last two decades, we have sounded the alarm about error in healthcare. We have talked about how healthcare workers do not wash their hands, about fires occurring in operating rooms, about surgeons operating on the wrong side of a patient's body, about how patients leave the hospital with the wrong medications. Despite a whole lot of effort, all of those things are still occurring. And patients are fed up with these ongoing errors in hospitals. So hospitals will have to figure out what battleships and big restaurants already know how to do, to be highly reliable organizations that never, never make errors."

As the speaker continues, he flashes images of workers assembling airplanes, automobiles, and rockets on the screen behind him. It is like a wartime propaganda film. I lose interest and start flipping through the packet his assistant is distributing. Inside is a copy of one of Atul Gawande's *New Yorker* essays, "Big Med," about how healthcare will be saved by becoming like the aircraft carrier or the assembly-line restaurant. I always look forward to Gawande's essays, so I tune out the speaker and start reading.

In the essay, Gawande described a trip to the Cheesecake Factory during which he ordered "a beet salad with goat cheese, white-bean hummus and warm flatbread, and the miso salmon."[1] Pleasantly surprised by the meal, he asked a line cook how the kitchen prepared the 308 items on the dinner menu and the 124 beverage choices. The line cook told him that each chef followed recipes displayed on a computer monitor at his or her station. Each chef could quickly produce any meal on the menu and tweak it to a diner's specifications.

Gawande was impressed. The Cheesecake Factory had figured out how to provide delicious meals at affordable prices by training its chefs to produce them efficiently and to incorporate new items effectively into the restaurant's ever-changing menu. He argued that medicine should follow suit. The training of today's physicians is both inefficient—a disjointed series of lectures, apprenticeships, and continuing medical education conferences—and ineffective, resulting in inconsistent patient outcomes. Sometimes physicians are like chefs who make beautiful meals but do not know how to get the dinner to the table at the right time for the right price, and sometimes they are like chefs who hastily deliver economical but unappetizing slop.

As I sat pondering Gawande's analogy, I wondered whether a restaurant that served beet salad with goat cheese offered the best analogy for the kind of medicine Gawande was advocating. Curious, I looked up the Cheesecake Factory's menu. So many meals, garlanded with so many adjectives. Baja Chicken Hash. Giant Belgian Waffle. Jamaican Black Pepper Shrimp. Sunrise Fiesta Burrito. Famous Factory Meatloaf. It was this last that struck me as a more fitting representation of what Gawande and the basement speaker wanted for medicine. Ordering the more fashionable-sounding beet salad missed the fact that if contemporary medicine is a meal, they were insisting that it be produced through industrial processes perfected at factories.

If Osler created a ladder for medical training—medical student to intern to resident to attending—then it was his contemporary, the legendary chef Auguste Escoffier, who created the comparable ladder for kitchens. It was Escoffier who codified the famous *brigade de cuisine* that characterizes a French haute cuisine kitchen. At the large hotels where Escoffier perfected the brigade system, a *maître de cuisine* oversaw several teams. Each team was headed by a chef who oversaw a particular portion of the meal: a *chef pâtissier* took charge of desserts, a *chef rôtisseur* the meat dishes, a *chef saucier* the sauces, a *chef entremetier* the soups and vegetable dishes, and a *chef poissonnier* the seafood. He even assigned a *chef garde-manger* to manage the pantry and a *chef de nuit* to operate the kitchen overnight.

In Escoffier's kitchen, each chef held his particular position for a time. A chef would spend months or years managing the pantry before learning to roast meats, prepare soups, or make sauces. Like Osler, Escoffier modernized his discipline by encouraging specialization and training. Through the process, a chef mastered the skills specific to each technique before becoming *maître de cuisine* of his own kitchen. Every chef learned every role. A person who invested time and energy in the kitchen departed with skills and with a new social role: master chef. In this way, Escoffier's kitchen was invested in transmitting the traditions of French cuisine by training apprentice chefs to be master chefs.

In addition to passing on the traditions of French cuisine and developing apprentices into masters, the brigade system was designed to enable the cooks to quickly prepare the meals ordered by a patron. According to Kenneth James's biography, Escoffier's "aim was for speed with quality. He achieved this by a production line technique where processes were carried out in parallel instead of sequentially, and each by a cook well-practised in his allocated procedure. [Escoffier] was able then to reduce the customers' waiting time to a minimum and to serve a quality dish at the right temperature."[2] Like Osler, Escoffier encouraged efficiency and effectiveness through the repetitive performance of a particular task.

The attending physician and the maître de cuisine were both men (or mostly men) who clambered up their professions' respective ladders by apprenticing themselves to more experienced practitioners. As they learned skills in these apprenticeships, they acquired the habits of the profession, and then, once they had completed their training, they transmitted those habits to students.

At first blush, the Cheesecake Factory sounds like a contemporary version of Escoffier's brigade. The Cheesecake Factory shares Escoffier's goal "to reduce the customers' waiting time to a minimum and to serve a quality dish at the right temperature." But the Cheesecake Factory is not a unique restaurant; it is a chain. The recipes at the Cheesecake Factory do not come from either the master chef or his or her subordinates in the brigade. The recipes come from corporate headquarters. Every six months, corporate headquarters introduces a new menu to match the fluctuating prices of food and the changing tastes of diners. For each dish, headquarters creates a script and then trains line chefs to follow the scripts. Less than a month after the new recipes are transmitted, line chefs are following the recipes and uniformly producing the meal designed at headquarters. The line chefs in this kitchen follow a corporate script rather than the counsel of a learned maître de cuisine.

Indeed, although the recipes are created by the corporation's chefs, the individual kitchens have no real maîtres de cuisine. In their place are kitchen managers looking over the shoulder of each line chef. If Escoffier's maître de cuisine was concerned with the quality of the meal, the Cheesecake Factory kitchen manager, according to Gawande, looks for waste and lost profit. For the kitchen manager to achieve the efficient results demanded by the Cheesecake Factory requires, in Gawande's words, "control, and they'd figured out how to achieve it on a mass scale."[3]

Control on a mass scale.

Quality-improvement advocates such as the basement speaker and Atul Gawande believe that the only way to fix healthcare is through controlling the practice of medicine on a mass scale. Healthcare is the largest industry in the United States, so we must use economies of scale to drive down costs and improve quality.

Most contemporary healthcare reform debates thus revolve around who controls healthcare, and the controllers are always conceived as some version of the market or the state. One side argues that government payers should mandate the care provided to patients. The other side argues that the market should determine what care is provided to patients. The genius of Gawande is that he split the difference, finding, in the kitchen of a casual dining restaurant, a happy synthesis of government regulations and market forces that he believed could work in healthcare. Just as the government regulates the production, preparation, and sale of food to ensure safety, it can regulate industrialized healthcare to protect patient safety. The market would determine what should be served, and the state would regulate its safety.

In this analogy, hospitals learn from chain restaurants to deliver innovative care to the most people possible for the least amount of money. Hospitals, like the Cheesecake Factory, could be improved if administrators studied best practices, standardized those practices, and then implemented them. Gawande argued that while physicians often know what the best practices are (such as those vetted by the Cochrane Collaboration), and even how to standardize them, they struggle when it comes to implementing them. It often takes physicians decades to introduce innovative practices into medicine; the Cheesecake Factory line chefs can master new recipes in days. Medicine, claimed Gawande, must be similarly standardized.

To illustrate the benefits of standardization, Gawande described how a private investment firm transformed six faltering hospitals by implementing "large-scale, production-line medicine" in their Intensive Care Units by combining bedside care with remote monitoring.[4] In these units, physicians and nurses at the bedside were like line chefs, while the physicians and nurses who remotely monitored the units were the kitchen managers. Describing a physician who remotely oversaw the units, Gawande wrote: "Ernst believes that his job is to make sure that everyone is collaborating to provide the most effective and least wasteful care possible." Ernst watched for errors—disconnected tubes, improper bed angles—and corrected them through video communication with the bedside staff. In Gawande's description, Ernst sounded less like one of Escoffier's maîtres de cuisine and more like a drone strike operator, a technician working at a bloodless remove from a deadly situation. The system Gawande described required bedside practitioners to perform, and remote practitioners to enforce, evidence-based standards of care. If this is what the future of medicine looks like, there will be bedside and remote physicians, just as there are kitchen managers and line chefs, but both kinds of physicians will work for the corporation that mandates the care the physicians do (and do not) deliver.

When we compare medicine to a standardized meal, we should ask what is lost in the process. Surely a meal can offer a very different experience to the patron even if it is prepared using the same ingredients, recipes, and techniques. Eating a beet salad prepared by a chef for restaurant patrons is a different experience from eating the same dish prepared for a potluck supper, a romantic meal shared by lovers, or an institutional meal served to prisoners, let alone a ritual meal like a familial Seder, a communal Iftar, or a prasada offering. The meals we eat have different meanings for us based on the occasions for which we prepare them and the people with whom we share them. When we focus on technique and outcomes, without concern for who prepares the meal for whom, the experience of the meals is neglected. Food becomes fuel.

When we extend this approach to the hospital and the clinic, the body is reduced to a collection of parts.

• • •

A neurosurgery resident is on the phone, apologizing for the call. He is requesting an ethics consult, and, as a member of our hospital's ethics committee, I answer his page. For the past decade, I have served on the ethics committees of the hospitals at which I have trained and worked. Sometimes we are consulted about difficult moral dilemmas, but most consults stem from a conflict between practitioners and patients, or their representatives, over when or whether to perform a medical intervention. The issues concern who controls the body, often a body in an Intensive Care Unit like those Ernst supervises.

"You can't do anything, I know, but my attending made me call," the neurosurgery resident says wearily. "It's hopeless. She is brain-dead on a blower, but I've talked to the family and they just don't understand. We're going to have to do the procedure anyway." I reassure him that he was right to call, and I ask the patient's name.

Tihun.

Tihun is a fifty-nine-year-old grandmother and Ethiopian immigrant. Several months before the consult, she was at home, watching three of her grandchildren while her daughters worked. Tihun suffered from a dull headache, but then the ache enveloped her. She began sweating and breathing heavily. She told her granddaughter she was struggling to stay awake. When the ambulance arrived, the paramedics found Tihun unconscious on her daughter's couch. Indeed, since the moment she lay down on the couch, Tihun had never regained full consciousness.

Sometime that afternoon, Tihun had suffered a hemorrhage of her pons, a portion of the brain that bridges the cerebrum and cerebellum. When the pons is damaged, it is a struggle to breathe, hear, move, sleep, and taste. For Tihun, the damage left her in a persistent vegetative state, a euphemism for a condition in which a person is awake but not aware.

The neurosurgery resident believed Tihun would die soon. How soon? He could not say, but he believed that further treatment would be meaningless. Tihun's daughters, on the other hand, wanted the neurosurgeons to place a permanent shunt, a sterile plastic drain, in the ventricles of Tihun's brain. When cerebrospinal fluid built up in her brain, the shunt would relieve the excessive fluid her body could no longer remove on its own. When I asked the resident about the shunt, he told me, "It's futile. The shunt won't affect her function. She has zero chance at meaningful further existence."

I asked to meet with the daughters. Through an interpreter, we sat down together in the break room on the surgical floor. They had never talked with their mother about what she would want done in this situation, but they did recall that Tihun would comment, "As long as there is life, there is hope," which they took to mean that she would want to remain alive. Neither daughter had much medical experience or had ever seen anyone die. What they had seen was the effects of a shunt. The daughters said that earlier in the week the neurosurgery team had proposed a permanent shunt to replace a temporary shunt that had reduced Tihun's agitation and pain. Throughout the conversation, they used the word *pressure* again and again, saying, "We want her to feel less pressured." To her daughters, the shunt relieved pressure on Tihun's brain. That was, after all, what the physicians had told them it would do. Her daughters also claimed that Tihun seemed different when the shunt was placed. They said she was "less pressured," and thus more able to be comforted by her family. They found this change meaningful.

They had known Tihun's maternal attention and affection, and they told me, "We want to care for her as she cared for us." I asked if they could recognize a difference between Tihun's maternal care and our invasive medical treatments. They could not.

I could sympathize with Tihun's daughters, who loved their mother and wanted to repay her affection by caring for her. But I could also sympathize with the neurosurgeon. I wished he had not suggested a procedure he believed would be futile. He had recognized, belatedly, a difference between caring for someone and performing a meaningless surgical procedure.

Seeing Tihun reminded me of when I was a medical student on the surgery services. I was forever getting caught up in the existential questions raised by illness, the disparate ways a person was altered by entering, through injury or illness, into the kingdom of the ill. Most of the surgeons I met were devoted, disciplined, and disinclined to take up such questions. They focused on body parts and wanted to talk about procedures—how to close a patent ductus arteriosus or to complete a living donor liver transplant, not what to meant to close a hole in one person's heart or to take a portion of one person's liver and place it another person's abdomen.

Quality-improvement experts can tell us the best way to complete both procedures. This, the accumulation of a century of learned effort, is a mighty achievement. Using the scientific spirit Osler summoned, the epidemiological rigor Cochrane championed, and the operational efficiency Deming routinized, today's quality-improvement experts design protocols and techniques for operationalizing our best practices from evidence-based documents like Cochrane reviews, turning several-hundred-page summaries into processes as clear as those displayed on the computers of line chefs at the Cheesecake Factory.

In their inability to answer the questions of either the neurosurgery resident or Tihun's daughters, though, we find a limit to what quality-improvement experts can do, to their claims to improve patient outcomes by displacing the subjective judgment of physicians with objective, evidence-based guidelines. In Tihun's case, those guidelines would help the surgical team place the shunt as efficiently and effectively as possible. But the quality-improvement experts cannot explain what it means for Tihun, her family, and those who care for her to keep her in a persistent vegetative state. This kind of life/ nonlife is possible only through contemporary medicine's technological control of the body, and no one knows how to define the meaning of such a life. Or how we can reconcile our furious efforts to keep Tihun alive with our anger at her daughters for wanting the very medical procedures we offer them.

Gawande characterized the meals at the Cheesecake Factory as "sweeter, fattier, and bigger" than necessary, but he and other quality-improvement advocates insist that Cheesecake Factory– style standardization is the solution to the healthcare system's ills.[5] Medicine, they say, is a series of procedures, scientifically informed techniques, that physicians provide to healthcare consumers. The pressing problems with medicine are not that it cannot answer the questions of Tihun's daughters or her physicians but that it is unable to deliver technical advances reliably enough. The solution therefore lies in delivery models that increase the medical profession's ability to innovate, to provide ever-better procedures ever more efficiently.

In this model, each physician becomes a technician, with a specific role to play in an industrial process. If we accept Gawande's analogy, we accept that we renew hospitals and clinics by turning them into factories where the physicians do not so much use a tool to encourage a patient's healing as engage a patient in an entire system of healthcare. I learned about this shift from tool to system from an interview with the philosopher Ivan Illich. I had not read Illich's work since medical school, when a professor recommended his landmark *Medical Nemesis*, which criticized contemporary medicine for medicalizing human existence.[6] Years later, in the last interviews he gave, Illich observed that what he had failed to recognize earlier in his career was that we have entered an era of "systems." Whereas we once used tools that were separate from their user, Illich said, we now engage with systems from which we perceive ourselves as inseparable. "In a system the user . . . becomes part of the system."[7] Instead of encouraging patients' ability to heal themselves, like a Hippocratic physician, or wielding a tool to affect the healing of a patient, like a nineteenth-century physician, the physicians of today, Illich concluded, are technicians who are inseparable from the systems in which they engage their patients.

So the line chef at a computer monitor or Ernst at his command center engage with the meal or the ICU patient only through the computer, and the computer is an instrument not of the chef or the physician but of the total system, the casual-dining restaurant or the chain hospital. Neither the chef nor Ernst can perform his or her task apart from the system. Unlike the earlier professionals who advanced through the hierarchies established by Escoffier and Osler, the chef and Ernst learn skills valued only within the system.

The authority that was once localized in the physician is dispersed throughout the healthcare system.

In such systems, Illich says the patient is conceptualized as "a system, that is, as an extraordinarily complex arrangement of feedback loops." The physician-technician perceives the patient as an inanimate, albeit complex, object to be controlled.

Illich's comment made me flip back through Gawande's essay. I wrote down all the things to which Gawande compared an ill person—a house on fire, a car, a solar panel, and a variety of meals—all inanimate objects. The restaurant analogy was actually harder to apply to medicine than it appeared: to the extent a patient requests a medical intervention, she or he is like a restaurant patron, but to the extent a patient is an object produced by a medical intervention, she or he is like the meal itself. Is an ill person the "product" of healthcare the way a meal is the product of a chef's work in the kitchen? A chef can manipulate the ingredients of a meal to whatever degree his or her skills allow, but by what should a physician's manipulation of the body be limited? How does this analogy take into account the needs of the patient and the ethical responsibilities of the physician? When we compare the ill to objects and declare the central question of medicine to be one of control, we reinforce the domination that Illich feared medicine exerts over them.

When we focus on outcomes—the ordered meal, prepared effectively and efficiently—over how and why the meal is prepared, we neglect the ways a process has meaning independent of its outcomes. That is another way in which restaurants are unlike hospitals. In a restaurant, you can always send back your overcooked plate of Famous Factory Meatloaf, and the kitchen will replace it with a new serving. In a hospital, the patient cannot ask for a new body. Patients have to live with the bodies with which they enter the hospital. Human bodies can be tinkered with, repaired sometimes, even improved on occasion, but cannot, finally, be fixed. We do a disservice to patients and their families when we suggest otherwise, when we encourage them to place their final hopes in medicine. The neurosurgery resident can either place or not place the shunt within Tihun's ventricles, he can relieve pressure or not, but the eventual outcome will still be her death. So sometimes how and why we care for the ill matters more than outcomes in hospitals.

Quality improvement enjoys support from hospitals, insurers, and regulators, but also from venture capitalists, tech evangelists, and corporate America.[8] The quality-improvement movement speaks to our technological utopian moment—how cool is it that we can re-fuel battleships in the ocean or that Ernst can monitor critically ill patients from thousands of miles away? But in turn it forces physicians and other practitioners to understand themselves as technicians instead of artisans. They are Ernst rather than Osler, line chefs rather than Escoffier, users of a system rather than wielders of a tool. So physicians have to abandon traditional ethical models intended for artisans and embrace the ethics of technicians. The ethical model of artisans is often called "virtue ethics," which makes it sound like training for Victorian-era prudery. But virtue ethics is not about sex, it is about how we form habits through relationships. In a virtue ethics account of medicine, a physician learns virtues like curiosity, humility, and patience through apprenticeships to excellent, experienced physicians. In today's ethical account of physicians, they are first and foremost efficient and effective technicians, inseparable from the system under which they work. So we develop systems and scripts with reliable outcomes instead of virtuous people who care for patients.

Systems work best in a world of quickly assembled (and disassembled) teams, and they encourage transient connections between these teams. If you work in one of today's medical factories, you often do not know which patients you will see on a given day. If you are superstitious, you might believe that full moons draw, like ill tides, waves of peculiar patients. If you are cynical, you might believe that the waning days of the month bring dependents whose government checks have been drunk away. If you are exhausted, you might believe that your very presence attracts the most demanding drug-seekers.

Whatever you believe, you care for the patients on your clinic schedule, census sheet, and sign-out list, along with whoever else gets
added to the queue.

If you work in one of today's medical factories, you also often do
not know who will work alongside you. Some days, I work with students from two or three disciplines, professionals from four or five
disciplines, and multiple physicians. Even on days when I see patients alone, I speak with social workers, nurses, various therapists,
and consulting physicians. We build and disassemble teams throughout a hospital day.

And just as the kitchen staff and the dining room patrons are
strangers to each other, so too in hospitals, where teams of strangers
prepare treatments for patients who are mostly unknown to us. We
know our patients as the MI in five, the UTI in seven, and the SI in
nine. They know us only because the nurses write our names on the
board above their beds. We know the patients as a myocardial infarction, a urinary tract infection, or a suicide attempt. Even our names
written above the bed are a kind of deceit: in a single day in a contemporary hospital, the physician responsible for a patient's care can
change with each shift. So to stay organized, physicians are learning to follow processes perfected by restaurants that have learned to
handle the problem of strangers preparing food for strangers.

Of course, complex processes rely upon an individual practitioner's
ability to tinker in the face of unanticipated events. The chef needs to
be able to tinker with a recipe when the tomatoes are overripe or the
fruit is sour. Physicians likewise need to tinker with evidence-based
scripts, and they have to be trained to figure out when and how to do
so. The ability to tinker, to adapt to changing circumstances, is hard
to account for in industrial processes focused on consistency, but in
virtue ethics tinkering is easily accounted for through the virtuous
habits of attentiveness to detail and flexibility, habits we cultivate
through life in a community. Even the best-engineered processes depend on these habits in their practitioners. But quality-improvement
advocates claim that well-engineered industrial processes actually
cultivate virtuous habits—they describe the wisdom of group ratio-

nality as embodied in industrial processes. And so physicians and other practitioners are being asked to learn not only our skills but also our ethics from participating in industrial-scaled systems.

But when the neurosurgeon resident pages me about Tihun, it is an implicit acknowledgment that the ethics of this system are inadequate. The neurosurgeons had done everything they were supposed to do according to the quality-improvement literature. They took a careful history from Tihun's daughters. They used an interpreter. When they finally agreed to the surgery on which the daughters insisted, they completed two separate checklists before making an incision. During the operation, they counted surgical instruments and pads to ensure they left none behind in Tihun's body. The operation was as efficient and as effective as the preparation of a meal in a corporate kitchen, but the surgeons operated with gritted teeth. Afterward, the resident again characterized the procedure as "meaningless" and Tihun's chances of "meaningful recovery at zero."

When I met with Tihun's daughters again after the permanent shunt was placed, they were pleased at the relief Tihun exhibited with less cerebrospinal fluid bearing down upon her brain, but they too were frustrated. They distrusted the surgeons. I asked whether they or Tihun trusted anyone to advise them about her health. They named the priest at their Ethiopian Orthodox church. They said he knew Tihun and understood what she wanted. They described Tihun as devout, making frequent appeals to God, as well to the Kidusan, a multitude of saints and angels who intercede with God on behalf of the faithful. I asked whether the physicians had ever spoken to the priest. The daughters shook their heads.

Tihun had a ladder as well, but it extended not up the line of a kitchen or the wards of a hospital but to her God. The neurosurgeons had involved Tihun's daughters, but not her priest, the Kidusan, or her God. They never figured out what being ill and receiving medical care meant to Tihun and her family.

Quality-improvement advocates rarely entertain the possibility that traditions outside the restaurant might have something to say about what we should eat and why—the possibility that instead of avoiding unwanted fuels, carbs, sugar, fat, or gluten, someone might want to avoid food that is treif or haram or contains the five pungent spices, food prohibited, respectively, in Judaism, Islam, and Buddhism. Similarly, the industrial hospital rarely considers that the traditions of health and illness and medicine embodied in Judaism, Islam, or Buddhism, with their millennia of wisdom, might teach us about processes relevant to good medical care. But this is perhaps more of a coup than an oversight. Foucault observed that in Western society, medicine replaced the cultural role of the church—displacing salvation with health and priests with physicians—but maintained its moral obligation. In the medieval era, we sought salvation; in the modern era, we are obligated to seek constant improvements in medical performance. We now believe suffering is bad itself, so we are morally obligated to eliminate pressure and pain. We physicians reduce pain simply to minimize it.

Foucault showed that we no longer allow alternative interpretations of the body. The body is interpreted by medicine or by the powers of modernity that it serves—the market or the state—not by the family or members of the synagogue, mosque, or temple. So the quality-improvement movement proposes to renew medicine within itself, by reducing adverse events, improving outcomes, and saving lives, without ever pausing to ask why we pursue health or to what end we seek to prevent death. When alternative interpretations of the body are disallowed, medicine circumscribes morality because it controls the only goods that we pursue: the elimination of suffering and the perfection of the body. Health is the good, so our pursuit of health for its own sake becomes the focus of our lives. Indeed, our lives become the avoidance of death. We resist death to resist death.[9] Or, returning to the restaurant analogy, we eat to eat.

In our new world of medicine, life consists of parts in motion, and medicine's job is to keep those parts moving. We die when a clot ruptures and occludes blood supply to our brain. That is all physicians can see. When we see the body today, it becomes an object that can be controlled and disciplined by medicine for the benefit of the market or the state. We see what happened to our bodies, not what our bodies mean as we live, love, and labor with our family, friends, and communities. We can no longer see the deep patterns of our bodies or their ultimate meaning. I am not sure Tihun's daughters could, either. While they invoked Tihun's faith, they were also the ones who requested the shunt. They were pursuing the relief of Tihun's pain with limited regard for what it would mean to Tihun's life. Tihun's daughters seemed obviously distinct from the neurosurgeon—by gender, ethnicity, and faith—but they were already part of the system. They wanted to order off the hospital's menu. They wanted to decide for Tihun.

In contemporary medicine, ethical conflicts are reduced to considerations of who decides, who chooses, and who orders what for whom. Someone has to choose, so questions of choosing, of control, are the only questions we ask. The Cheesecake Factory offers many options, but the limitation is that you have to pick something from the menu, and you are not encouraged to ask why you should eat it or what it means to eat all that food.

Of course, the most recent trend in restaurants is to emphasize the authentic, local, and particular. The garlic scapes are grown behind the restaurant. The chef forages for the morels. The eggs were laid that morning by the restaurant's prize hens. The particularity of each ingredient, each chef, is celebrated. Every time I go to work, though, the hospital is celebrating the consistency of its production. The infection rate beats the national average. The surgical suite is set up according to international guidelines. The physicians are assessed through Press Ganey scores. The uniformity of each procedure, each provider, is celebrated. I wonder why we are moving away from standardization in our restaurants and toward it in our hospitals.

Instead of altering medicine so it can serve the complex meals only an industrial process can produce, we could call on medicine to serve simple suppers. Instead of calling on physicians to become line chefs or kitchen managers in an industrial process, we could call on them to be, like farm-to-table chefs, rooted in the particularities, the terroir, of a local community. We could reinvigorate the guild model and its model of the physician as an artisan who carefully passes on accumulated wisdom. Just as some food writers suggest teaching people to cook at home rather than to eat out, we could empower patients to choose healthy habits as a way to practice self-care.

The American government currently has more than a dozen different agencies measuring the quality of medical care. Insurers, accrediting agencies, and licensing boards have their own measures as well. Together, they are pushing medicine toward uniform outcomes, with little acknowledgment of the particularities of people and places. The goal of standardization does not recognize that excellence can be achieved in many different ways—Ethiopian cuisine should not be like the food at the Cheesecake Factory. It took us decades to pivot away from the standardization of food, and someday we may shift our focus away from the standardization of medicine.

For now, though, we are eating Famous Factory Meatloaf. It is efficiently and effectively prepared fuel, but it is not a meal. For a true meal, you need other people with whom to share the food and a culture of preparing, serving, and sharing food. Beyond bare quality improvement, we need to cultivate a culture of health that addresses the analogous questions of what it means to be well, to be ill, and to seek and provide medical assistance. We need a way out of the factory.

nine

Connie was sure her sister was plotting against Peyton Manning. She wanted to warn him, so she would yell, "Peyton, Peyton, watch out, she is coming for you!" when she woke up and as she collapsed into sleep. Her warnings went unanswered, so she knocked over a chair at her nursing home and threatened to keep knocking over chairs until the Denver Broncos' star quarterback visited her. She needed to know he was safe. The overworked staff at her nursing home tried to soothe her, to redirect her, and to ignore her. Finally, they called a social worker from our hospital for an evaluation.

When he arrived, Connie was shouting threats. Having tried unsuccessfully to calm her, he placed her on a mental health hold, a form of involuntary psychiatric treatment. The sheriff transported Connie to our Emergency Room, where the on-call physician interviewed her. The physician had never met Connie and had no access to any records of her care, yet he was responsible for determining whether she had a mental illness and if, as a result of that illness, she was dangerous to herself or others. He diligently documented what he heard—Connie was threatening to kill her sister to save Peyton Manning's life—and Connie's fate was sealed: involuntary hospitalization on the psych unit.

I work every day on the unit, so I can tell you that real-life psych units bear little resemblance to the dimly lit places run by syringe-wielding sadists you see in the movies. Most resemble rented space at an office park. The modular carpeting is dark enough to hide the occasional stain. The walls are painted in muted earth tones and decorated with framed reproductions of soothing landscapes. When you look more closely, though, you can see signs that this building houses something other than business executives. Our framed pictures are bolted to the wall with recessed screws. Our windows are triple-paned and sashless, fixed in place. Our doors are locked with antiligature pull handles. You cannot take these pictures off the wall or open these windows. You cannot walk out these doors without a physician's order.

The morning after Connie was admitted, I arrived on the unit and read her chart. She sounded dangerous and threatening. Then I saw her, a seventy-two-year-old kyphotic woman rounded over herself like a collapsed star, shuffling along a curved path with the assistance of a cane. She muttered that her older sister Rhonda would get to Peyton today. She begged us to call Peyton and warn him.

I did not know how to get Peyton's phone number, so I asked Connie for Rhonda's instead. When we called, Rhonda's daughter told us that Rhonda had been dead for twenty years. If Rhonda posed a threat to Peyton Manning, he would need an exorcist, not a physician.

The report we got about Connie was simple: she had a long history of schizophrenia. We assumed, therefore, that she had experienced a recurrence after refusing her medication at the nursing home. Association slipped into causation, and the story was complete: Connie was psychotic because she was refusing medications.

I have learned to distrust completed stories, though, so I decided to approach Connie differently. She would not tolerate a full physical examination, but I found that she would walk with me and let me to listen to her heart and lungs as long I allowed her to remain upright. When Connie stood, she shook like a wind-blown tree, and something about her movement reminded me of a history book I had recently read.

The book, *Rooted in the Earth, Rooted in the Sky: Hildegard of Bingen and Premodern Medicine*, described the medical practice of Hildegard of Bingen, a medieval abbess. Despite her cloistered existence, Hildegard was a polymath who, in addition to working as an abbess, musician, mystic, and theologian, was also a gardener and an infirmarian who cared for the ill in her community's infirmary. When the book's author, a medical historian and physician named Victoria Sweet, analyzed the practical manuals written by Hildegard, she found that Hildegard's infirmary, a sick house where the ill were diagnosed and treated, included an herb garden where Hildegard could grow medications and a pharmacy where she could compound them. Hildegard was equally at home in the clinic and the garden, and she tended ill bodies and ill plants with the same care.[1]

As I examined Connie, my wind-blown patient, I wondered what treatment I would give her if I emulated Hildegard and acted as a physician-gardener.

• • •

Victoria Sweet's second book, *God's Hotel: A Doctor, a Hospital, and a Pilgrimage to the Heart of Medicine*, recounts her own attempts to adopt a version of Hildegard's practice. In the memoir, Sweet described practicing medicine at Laguna Honda, a public almshouse dedicated to rehabilitation and skilled nursing services for a diverse and underserved population in San Francisco. Most of her patients were impoverished and cycled in and out of area hospitals whenever they experienced an acute crisis. Every time they were admitted to area hospitals, they were treated according to the evidence-based algorithms of industrial medicine. They always received life-saving care. They were also always discharged back to the streets of San Francisco. In those inhospitable environs, their health inevitably deteriorated, and they were hospitalized again to start the cycle anew.

As a physician at a safety-net hospital for the urban underserved, I see this cycle every day. Patients are stabilized in the hospital, discharged to places where they cannot maintain their health, and return within weeks or months. Sensing a kindred spirit, I eagerly read Sweet's memoir.

Sweet observed that when people grow ill, they enter hospitals whose purpose and architecture were defined hundreds of years before germ theory and the discovery of the genome. When people receive care as patients or work in these hospitals as practitioners, Sweet showed, they unknowingly follow scripts written by our premodern predecessors. Sweet had trained as historian, so she could see the premodern scripts underlying our contemporary hospitals as if they were "shadow texts that could sometimes be discerned beneath another text."[2] Sweet wanted patients and practitioners to bring some of these premodern texts out of the shadows, out of the recesses of our thoughts and desires. She wanted us to reclaim them for our daily use.

To do so, Sweet engaged Hildegard's concept of *viriditas*. Hildegard understood all of her seemingly disparate activities as unified under this Latin word, which means, literally, "greening." For Hildegard, viriditas is always a divine gift, the invigorating force of life that animates the body just as sap animates a tree. Without viriditas, the human body is mere matter, either inert or decaying, like a plant without sap. As this simile suggests, Hildegard understood the sickbed and the garden bed as analogues of each other. Viriditas animated both human beings and plants, and therefore both could be healed by its renewal. So Hildegard tended to the ill in her infirmary as she cared for the plants in her community's garden—by observing the environment in which a patient's body was situated, removing the obstacles to the renewal of viriditas, and encouraging the body's ability to heal by giving, say, less or more food, drink, or rest.

Sweet so admired Hildegard's approach that she put it into practice at Laguna Honda. As Sweet followed Hildegard's model of looking for ways to repair or strengthen the viriditas of her patients, she noticed a change in the way she approached them. Instead of acting like a technician searching for the broken part to fix or replace, she began encouraging the self-healing of her patients, as a gardener would encourage her plants.

As she began approaching patients like a gardener, she found renewed meaning in the practice of medicine. She found a medicine in which "the body was not imagined as a machine nor disease as a mechanical breakdown," and the physician could appreciate the wonders and mysteries of the bodies of her patients.[3] Sweet argued that while a physician-technician looked for fixes—I thought of treating herniated discs with discectomy, obesity with gastric-bypass surgery, or rapid mood swings with mood stabilizers—a physician-gardener helped a patient resolve these illnesses organically. A physician-gardener might advise learning new habits over time, like daily stretching, dietary changes, and coping strategies.

After adopting some of Hildegard's practices, Sweet also found that her perception of time changed. And as her perception shifted, she stopped feeling frantic and alienated from her patients. Indeed, Sweet found that time itself was the critical ingredient in their care. She described one patient, Terry Becker, who needed two and a half years to be restored to health. Two and a half years is an eternity in today's hospitals, where efficiencies are celebrated.

Sweet knows this, knows the many obstacles to prescribing "tincture of time" in contemporary medicine. Administrators insist upon brief patient encounters that can be billed at the maximum level. Insurers demand rapid discharge. Regulators standardize care. There are many demands upon the time we physicians might like to give patients. When I spend more than the usual time with a patient, panic sometimes grows in my gut, as I worry about where these extra moments will have to be borrowed from the remainder of my day.

This is a shame, because Sweet is right: many patients are able to heal only when physicians give them a sufficient period of time to heal themselves in a supportive environment. There are, of course, pragmatic considerations, which Sweet acknowledged. For acute conditions like appendicitis, sepsis, or myocardial infarction, physicians should still act like efficient technicians. Remove the appendix, treat the infection, stent the heart. Fix the broken part. In chronic conditions, like the dull abdominal pain that presents six months post-appendectomy, the lingering fatigue following sepsis, or the vague depression after myocardial infarction, physicians should act like wise gardeners by prescribing watchful waiting and considered observation. Instead of rushing to diagnostic tests, imaging, and treatments, physicians should follow the patient over the seasons and cycles of time.

A version of medicine that depicted the body as a wonder rather than a machine: the physician as a gardener rather than as a technician, and the hospital as a garden rather than a factory. I found this vision entrancing.

After even a few years of seeing much, the practice of medicine becomes routine. You start to recognize patterns. One of the patterns

I see is a person with a known psychotic disorder who stops taking his or her meds and subsequently experiences psychosis. So the story the admitting physician told about Connie raised no eyebrows. Connie has schizophrenia, an often-devastating and progressive disorder that remains poorly understood, even though it affects 1 percent of the world's population and causes 10 percent of the world's disabilities. She has an extensive medical record that dates back to her first episode as an adolescent, and she has been in and out of psychiatric hospitals, and on and off medications for most of her life.

There are many ways to account for schizophrenia. One neuroscientific explanation is that it is a sensory-gating stimuli disorder, an inability to sift through the stimuli that surround us: the tastes of foods, the touch of other people, the sounds of the city, and all the other stimuli in our worlds. Most of us learn to filter through the various stimuli unconsciously and focus on a particular thing or a task at hand. People with schizophrenia often struggle to do so. They are unable to shut out a thought, a smell, a taste, a sight, or a sound that the rest of us can ignore as we go through our day.[4] When people with schizophrenia become paranoid, it usually means that they have overinterpreted some stimulus in their life. They might fear people they know or the environment in which they live or what they hear discussed. In the 1960s, people with schizophrenia were often paranoid about Communists. Today, they frequently fear terrorists and government surveillance or become obsessed with celebrities and athletes like, well, Peyton Manning.

In Denver, however, not just psychotics but rabid fans as well are obsessed with Peyton Manning. And while paranoia certainly occurs during a psychotic episode, it is a symptom of many ailments; it can also occur when a person is sleep-deprived, anxious, or taking (or withdrawing from) any number of licit and illicit drugs. Another trigger for paranoia can be delirium, and I wondered whether that could be the case with Connie. When people are delirious, they are confused, struggle to follow conversations, and have trouble navigating even familiar environments, let alone unfamiliar environments like a psychiatric ward. The irony is that when they most need a familiar, soothing environment, they are admitted to the purposeful bustle of a contemporary hospital, where the many movements and noises can be provocative.

• • •

Sometimes the assumptions we make through seeing much are wrong. Sometimes physicians overinterpret the available evidence. I suspected that we were fitting Connie's story into our expected patterns. So when I evaluated her, I decided to try something different, to engage her as if I were a gardener-physician.

I sat at the nursing station and watched Connie for a few minutes. I wanted to see how she moved through the room. She sat for a moment, rose from the chair, approached the nurses to say, "I lied," and then began organizing the chairs in an unhinged semicircle, as though they faced an unseen fire. As she moved, her gown flapped in the breeze, revealing her bare chest.

At this point, I decided to approach Connie, offering her a shirt to cover herself. She received it from me wordlessly, then stepped into the shirt's armholes as though it were another pair of pants. She was evidently confused, so I started over and introduced myself. I asked Connie her name. She knew it. She knew her birthdate as well. So I asked for that day's date. "Red." She struggled with memory, unable to remember a few common objects after a minute or two. She became irritable when I assessed her level of attention by asking her to spell a word backward. She could not name the president. I asked her to hold my finger and, as I spelled out a word, squeeze it whenever I said the letter A. Instead, she simply squeezed my hand every few seconds. Connie was paranoid to be sure, but she was also delirious.

The causes of delirium are numerous. Infection, dehydration, or various medications are common causes, and physicians have lists of questions to help them assess for each possibility, but Connie could not answer many questions, so we needed to examine her body for clues. As we examined her, I tried to envision her body as a storm-battered though once-sturdy tree. Was her problem in the bark (her mottled skin), the leaves (her brittle hair), or the branches (her de-conditioned limbs)? I looked for signs of past or present pests. Her glasses were crooked, her hair unkempt, and she favored her right foot. Her pants smelled of urine. Watching her gave me a few clues, and the gradual gathering of them had reassured Connie enough that she finally allowed us to sample her blood and urine for further study.

One solution for an ailing and tired-appearing patient like Connie would be to take the analogy between physicians and gardeners literally and prescribe Hildegard's herbal medicines. Some admirers of Hildegard take her medical manuals as recipe books rather than inspirations. They plant, compound, and consume the herbal preparations Hildegard described: fennel seeds to ease indigestion; lavender wine to increase understanding; aloe and myrrh to relieve headaches. The books dedicated to the literal reclamation of Hildegard's medicine are full of premodern generalizations. In one of those recipe books, I read, "People with green eyes are good craftsmen and very good at learning a new trade. Other characteristics include stability and cunningness."[5] As a green-eyed physician, I can be cunning, but I struggle to learn new trades. This kind of generalization explains little about me, but it reminds me of how much separates us from Hildegard.

Hildegard lived before Darwin, Newton, even Copernicus. She thought the position of the earth was settled in the sky and that the sun, moon, and stars rotated about the fixed earth. Their rotations generated not only time and the changing seasons, but the components of health and illness of plants and people alike. To reclaim Hildegard's medicine literally, you need more than a well-loved herb garden. You need premodern astrology and biology. But most practitioners of what is called contemporary and alternative medicine proffer treatments from the premodern garden without endorsing the premodern understanding of nature. Advocates chew fennel seeds but keep time like the rest of us, assuming that our planet rotates about the sun and that time can be exchanged for money.

Thinking of Connie as a tree was an inspiring analogy but not a useful recipe for her care.

• • •

Victoria Sweet does not encourage physicians to become herbalists who re-create the medicines Hildegard compounded. Sweet appreciates and employs contemporary allopathic medicines. What she wants is for contemporary physicians to prescribe their medications within a physician-patient relationship like those that Hildegard developed with her community members.

Contemporary physicians so often begin and end patient encounters with medications that healthcare executives often call physicians "prescribers." So when Connie visited her physician every three months at our local mental health center, the visit was aptly described as a "fifteen-minute med check" because the questions were all about the efficacy and adverse effects of the medications. Not so for Hildegard, who began the medical encounter with a careful observation of the patient, followed it with an examination, and only then might offer a prescription. Hildegard's prescriptions included both a regime and a medication designed to maintain (not simply restore) health. The regime encompassed rules for living that addressed the most healthful quantity and quality of emotion, exercise, food, and sleep, and it was personalized for each individual's humors, age, and climate. Hildegard's infirmary was no factory.

Sweet believed that contemporary physician-gardeners could also prescribe both a regime and a medication. Instead of simply prescribing a medication or performing a procedure—what physicians are encouraged to do by contemporary billing practices—physicians could modify a patient's internal and external environment to fortify his or her ability to heal. Instead of, say, prescribing olanzapine to a child who acts out, a physician-gardener would design behavioral and educational interventions and follow the child through his or her developmental stages. Instead of prescribing testosterone cream to a faltering man, a physician-gardener would help him improve his energy levels through exercise and rest. Instead of operating on aging knees, a physician-gardener would teach the patient ways to strengthen the muscles surrounding them. This might sound radically opposed to contemporary medical practices, but by the standards of evidence-based medicine, there is actually little reason to recommend antipsychotics to irritable children, testosterone to aging men, and knee surgeries to the middle-aged. There are, however, financial incentives for recommending each intervention. Sweet wanted to incentivize physicians differently so that, like Hildegard, they approached the body as a plant that could heal itself gradually, within realistic limits.

Yet Sweet developed her ideal at some remove from Hildegard's garden and infirmary. Sweet practiced in a contemporary hospital, while Hildegard lived in a premodern monastery. Sweet cared for the patients admitted to her service, while Hildegard cared for fellow members of her Benedictine community. In a cloistered community, the therapeutic alliance between physician and patient was established well before a medical relationship was initiated. They shared a common life and lived by a common rule; their common rhythm was a sung hymn.

Do we need to restore such communities or therapeutic alliances to reclaim hospitals as gardens instead of factories and make physicians gardeners instead of technicians? That would be a dramatic reconfiguration, but perhaps we can still work to reenchant medicine with some of the mystery that has been lost in the modern world.

Reading Sweet had reminded me of Max Weber's observation that our rational modern world, with our ability to generate evidence-based guidelines and standardize best practices, came at the cost of an enchanted view of the world. Premodern people, Weber wrote, understood the natural world as a mystery, governed by "mysterious incalculable forces" in which they participated.[6] When we perceive the world as made up of materials (including the body) that we can enumerate, manipulate, and control, Weber wrote, mystery and wonder are replaced by technical means and calculations. If we could reenchant medicine, perhaps we could move away from the model of physicians as technicians controlling the failing parts of a patient and allow them to be more like gardeners tending to patients. Physicians would understand themselves and their patients as part of the natural world that remains, for all our scientific knowledge, mysterious.

My training taught me to see the body as a machine made up of parts. I learned that physicians identify themselves by the part of the machine for which they are responsible. We are consulted when our part of a patient's body falters, and we sign off on the case when we cannot think of how to help that part further, even if the patient remains ill. We see the body as a collection of interrelated problems. We might say something like, "Connie has an infection in her urinary tract that has caused delirium in her brain." But there are at least two difficulties with that sentence.

The first difficulty is that by our own measures we struggle to understand why an infection in the bladder and kidneys could profoundly impair the brain. We believe that dehydration and shifts in essential minerals like sodium and potassium are involved. We know that neurotransmitters like acetylcholine and dopamine are altered. We believe that inflammatory cytokines are involved. We know that, in the year after developing delirium, 35–40 percent of patients will die. Yet all we can conclude is, as stated in a review article I read while caring for Connie, "The pathophysiology of delirium remains poorly understood."[7] We physicians struggle when the parts of the body are interrelated in complex ways.

The second difficulty is that it posits the body as primarily a problem. Reading Sweet, I thought of the poet Christian Wiman and his observation that "existence is not a puzzle to be solved but a narrative to be inherited, and undergone, and transformed person by person."[8] Given the limitations of our science, it seemed more apt to engage Connie's delirium as a narrative that could be transformed through a therapeutic relationship than to treat it as a disease and send her on her way.

• • •

We began with the fixes. She had too little potassium, so we ordered supplemental potassium. She had *E. coli* bacteria growing in her urine, so we administered an antibiotic. She was psychotic, so we ordered an antipsychotic.

Then we addressed her habits. Connie had become accustomed to taking medications for which we could find no indication, and we pruned them from her medication list. She was up all night, circling the unit in loops that never closed; we established clear times for being asleep and awake. She confused the date with the color red, so we oriented her each time we met her. Then we tried to form a therapeutic alliance with her, but Connie was not interested. She still wanted the Broncos rather than the shrink squad.

I wondered whether the only way to build a therapeutic alliance might be to provide literal enchantment. That ought to be easy in Colorado. The windows of our unit look out upon the Rocky Mountains erupting from the plains, but the steel safety wire cross-hatched into each pane of glass obscures the view. The view out those windows is encumbered rather than enchanted. The unit is, like a factory or an office park, designed for the standardized encounter, for safety, for efficiency. You have to work to find enchantment on the unit. Ours is a hospital for the poor, where a literal garden would be an unfunded luxury, an inefficient use of scarce space, a pretense—or a place where the methadone patients would sell their doses. Instead of a garden, we have a little landscaping near the entrance. It has flowers, a water feature, some bushes, and a few young trees, but the whole area takes up no more space than the backyard of a suburban home. Among the trees, emaciated girls from the eating disorder unit sit sullenly in their wheelchairs while trauma patients lean against the branches of their IV poles while balancing cigarettes between the yellowed fingers of bandaged hands. When I visit this space, I feel little enchantment. I wish we could give our patients more of the enchantment of the natural world—a garden, a forest, an expanse of green—but the cost is prohibitive. I have to translate Sweet and Hildegard, become a metaphorical gardener.

More often I feel like a factory farmer. The goal of commercial agriculture, like that of the healthcare industry, is to maximize yields. But the analogy breaks down when we think about what each industry is creating. Factory farmers can simply cull underperforming crops and focus their attention on the high-performing crops. We do not cull, but in the healthcare industry it is common to neglect the indigent ill in favor of healthy, well-insured patients. (When a neighborhood becomes impoverished, hospitals relocate to wealthier neighborhoods and call it an effort to change their "payer mix.")

I think Sweet is right that physicians are charged to care for the indigent ill—we cannot neglect these patients in favor of the healthy and well-insured—and it makes sense to understand a physician as more akin to a gardener than a factory farmer. But being a physician-gardener in today's hospital cannot mean copying Hildegard's recipe books and declaring that green-eyed people are cunning. It requires translation.

For Connie, the enchantment we could offer was the hospital's therapy dog. He proved remarkably effective. As Connie caressed his shaggy coat, her shoulders relaxed and her eyes cleared. She could sit still in his company. Despite her delirium, she had a capacity for joy in the presence of her fellow animal. He provided enough enchantment for her to form an alliance.

Sweet describes her proposal for medical reform as "slow medicine," an analogy to the slow food movement. At the same time that people are turning away from mass-produced and standardized food in favor of locally grown and craft-produced meals, Sweet wants physicians to turn away from standardized medicine. Reading Sweet, I thought back to my reservations about Famous Factory Meatloaf and tried to imagine a medical practice that adopted some of the commitments of the farm-to-table and locavore food movements. Could the practice of medicine be particular to specific places and seasons?

When we hear about variations in medical care, it is usually in the form of a criticism, identifying a deviation from the norm. The most trenchant criticism comes from the *Dartmouth Atlas of Health Care*. The atlas combines zip code–level records of Medicare claims overlaid onto a finely detailed map of the United States. With the click of a few buttons, you can find out how the rate of particular surgical procedures, the availability of physicians, or the use of prescription drugs varies across a state or region. The *Atlas's* intuitive graphical interface makes it easy to access data that were previously squirrelled away in a thousand government records. It is startling to see how much variation occurs and how the key variant appears to be whether a particular service is available. If physicians can profitably perform a medical intervention for the patients in their zip code, they seem to do so, irrespective of the medical necessity of the intervention. The curators of the *Atlas* rightly describe it as a critical tool for improving "understanding of the efficiency and effectiveness of our health care system" and note that "this valuable data forms the foundation for many of the ongoing efforts to improve health and health systems across America."[9] In their description, they situate the *Atlas* as a worthy advance in Cochrane's reorientation of medicine around effectiveness and efficiency on the population level. And, as in Cochrane's work, the *Atlas* describes variations in care as inefficiencies to be identified and eliminated.

I admire the editors' aim, but worry that the *Atlas* neglects other kinds of regional variations, some of which seem desirable to me. Who wants every place to feel like no place at all? In medical school, I met physicians who belonged specifically to North Carolina. They had grown up, trained, and practiced in the area. They had courtly manners and uncommon names. Axalla Hoole. Georgette Dent. Jacob Lohr. Their accents were as particular as their commitment to the Goodliest State and its research university. As physicians and teachers, they listened to stories and told stories. When students joined Jacob Lohr's service, he asked them to tell a story. You belonged to his team if you could tell a story well. Physicians like Jacob Lohr moved slowly but with purpose.

The best physicians share this ability to form a relationship with a patient that develops into a story. The first time I saw a child with failure to thrive for an unknown reason, I could not get the child to stay still long enough for an examination. But Jacob Lohr asked a few questions of the child's parents, played a small game with a child, and got him or her to relax so that he could perform the examination.

By the end of an encounter, the examined child would be calm, the parents charmed, and Lohr had integrated all the known information into a narrative diagnosis and prescription. The parents thanked him, and I stood in the corner, wondering how he did it.

Since Lohr never acted like a technician following a script, when he attended on the wards the hospital felt more like Hildegard's garden than like a factory for the efficient diagnosis and treatment of disease. Time did not press upon him, but was rather part of the treatment. Lohr would sit with patients. Listen to their stories. Communicate his findings and counsel in stories of his own. His service was a master class in forming therapeutic relationships. So now, when I see patients like Connie, I call upon the craft I learned from physicians like Dr. Lohr. I look for a story we can share.

Hospitals often post quotations from Osler, but consultants write our slogans.

Halfway through residency, a new CEO took over the C suite at the academic medical center in Chapel Hill. Like the owner of a new home, he gave the place a makeover. He hired consultants to interview employees, organize focus groups, and compare the hospital's outcomes with those of peer institutions. The consultants recommended that we increase high-margin procedures, eliminate low-margin services, and rebrand the hospital. Consultants wrote a new marketing slogan to describe the plan and organized meetings for each department at which they informed us of our future and announced the slogan that embodied it. At the end of each meeting, assistants offered attendees a T-shirt with the hospital's new slogan on the front in block letters. Then the consultants flew home.

The T-shirts sat in boxes, uncollected. In the subsequent weeks, the hospital kept offering the free T-shirts to employees. At four in the morning, I would be five patients behind in the emergency department, my pager going off every few moments while ill people sobbed to themselves behind thick doors. A voice, like that of an unnamed minor divinity, would suddenly come from the loudspeaker in the ceiling. "All employees are invited to the second floor to collect their free T-shirt and show their pride in our hospital's mission." I never saw anyone leave a bedside or nursing station to get a shirt; the nurses and physicians were all firmly harnessed to the heavy carts of patient care.

The T-shirts were dumped in the hospital's surplus clothes closets. A few weeks later, I started noticing them on rehab patients on the eighth floor, then on ward patients on the fourth floor. The shirts seemed to be making their way down the stairs of the hospital's bed towers floor by floor. It was only a matter of time before they got to the psych unit on the third floor.

I saw them appear one Monday morning when I arrived at the psychotic ward, an eighteen-bed unit where most of the patients were being held involuntarily. We had several new admissions. Most of the new patients were wild-eyed and ranting. Some were hollow-eyed and shuffling. Some wore their own clothes. But others wore the new T-shirts, with the consultants' slogan across their chests: "I'M COMMITTED!"

I think of those T-shirts and their unintentional insult when I sit through yet another presentation from a consultant about how to transform medicine by adopting disruptive and innovative techniques. They use peppy slogans, folksy anecdotes, and passive-aggressive dicta such as, "If you don't like change, you're going to like irrelevance even less." (I often fantasize about asking them to speak that way to our patients.) The consultants are not fluent speakers of the language of medicine. Their native tongue is business, and they often describe the hospital as another industrial site that should respond to the kind of industrial practices that work in factories. They describe patients as consumers and physicians as providers of healthcare services. But describing us as providers misses the role that physicians—as well as nurses, pharmacists, social workers, and other medical practitioners—still have as craftsmen and women.

I never hear consultants or basement speakers describe medicine as a craft, but some of the old physicians still walking the floors of the hospital will pull me aside at staff meetings or at the nurse's station late on a Saturday evening to talk about it that way. They appreciate the way science was used to inform medicine after Flexner's *Report*, but confide that medicine used to be something more than a job, even something more than a profession. They "practiced" medicine because they were always improving their craft and passing it along to the next generation. Like carpenters or bricklayers, they traveled about as journeymen, seeking experience in their craft. They found a master, apprenticed themselves to the master, and became, with effort, masters themselves. These old physicians remember the first morning they scrubbed in on a thoracotomy, the evenings they spent practicing their sutures on a scrap piece of beef begged from the butcher, and the year they learned to replace joints alongside an august physician. They accreted experiences while slowly, repetitiously developing their craft. These old physicians tell the stories of when physicians were craftsmen and women who learned from master physicians instead of from standardized curricula or datasets or market trends. Wisdom was won, was earned—not derived. These old physicians disliked slogans, but they loved to share a maxim or two that they had learned from their masters, maxims that had guided their practice of medicine.

These maxims referred to the many prudential judgments a physician makes in a day, never to the biostatistical measures that evidence-based medicine advocates designed to guide clinical practice—no Number Needed to Treat or Number Needed to Harm, as measured in the Cochrane reviews—but practical reasoning for determining the best action when confronted by competing options.

Common things are common. When you hear hoofbeats, think horses not zebras.

Local pain is a danger. Widespread pain is a bother.

Think twice, cut once.

Heal with steel.

All bleeding eventually stops.

Good judgment comes from experience. Experience comes from poor judgment.

Many of these maxims relate to surgical practice, presumably because surgeons take the risks of going beneath the body's surface. In our own way, psychiatrists are also interested in what lies beneath the surface. Yet we engage the intimate details in different ways. Psychiatrists probe by means of questions, silences, and suggestions. Surgeons probe with hands, scalpels, and scopes. Like us, they sometimes err when they probe, so they think a lot about mistakes and how to prevent them.

At the hospital where I trained, many of the surgeons wore cloisonné owl pins on the lapels of their white coats. The pins intrigued me because they looked like they belonged on the naphthalene-perfumed coats of elderly symphony-goers, not on the priestly coats of surgeons, and I could not figure out the pattern of their distribution. I saw the pins on attending surgeons and chief residents and, on occasion, on the coat of a surgical intern.

Finally, I asked a surgical resident, "What's the deal with the owl pins? They make you look like my grandmother."

"You get one for taking out a healthy appendix."

"What? Why would you be rewarded for removing a healthy organ? Is this like handing out ribbons for surgical sadist of the week?"

"No. The idea is that appendicitis can be so deadly that it is better to remove a healthy appendix than to miss a ruptured appendix."

"Oh. So why the owl?"

He sighed, exasperated at the incessant questions.

"The owl is a symbol of wisdom, of making the right decision, the wise choice—it's better to save a life and lose an appendix than to save an appendix and lose a life."

His old-lady pin was really a merit badge.

• • •

The idea of rewarding wisdom, encouraging a physician to develop prudential judgment, is in disrepute. Cochrane and the pioneers of evidence-based medicine disliked the ways it relied upon anecdotal evidence: miss one ruptured appendix and you are likely to take out a hundred healthy appendixes. Today's quality-improvement advocates dislike the way that prudential judgment leads patients through unstandardized scripts to inconsistent outcomes. In the same hospital, different surgeons have very different rates of appendectomies. Multiplied over a population, startling differences in surgical rates occur.

Both concerns have obvious merit. Both concerns also neglect the ongoing need of physicians to make wise judgments.

Physicians need to exercise judgment in applying evidence-based literature to a specific patient. Even if you have mastered the best evidence, you still have to know how to curate, integrate, and apply the evidence to the patient before you, especially since there is often limited evidence available that applies to a specific patient.

On the psych unit, we suffer this problem every day. The acute treatment of persons with schizophrenia usually includes a medication to reduce the symptoms of psychosis. There are many randomized clinical comparison trials of the various antipsychotics. These trials, however, typically exclude persons who also abuse substances or who have unstable living situations. The former confuses the effect of the treatment, and the latter makes it hard for participants to finish a study protocol. But the result is that we have to extrapolate from the populations in clinical trials to the patients in front of us, who are often more ill and more impoverished than the more stable subjects who populate the evidence-based literature.

A few months ago, Doreen was the patient in front of us, fresh off the bus from New Mexico. We admit ill travelers like Doreen daily because most counties in the state, even in the surrounding states, have no psychiatrist. People who need to see a shrink have to come to Denver. The city sits at the foot of the Rocky Mountains and at the intersection of two interstate highways. I-25 runs vertically along the Rockies most of the way from Canada to Mexico. I-70 travels horizontally, spanning much of the distance from the Pacific to the Atlantic. When a passenger becomes manic or psychotic on a bus, the driver is encouraged to keep the passenger on board until the bus, whether it has to traverse mountain passes or the eastern plains, can stop in Denver.

Doreen ran onto the bus in Las Cruces, still tweaking on meth, collapsed into sleep before Albuquerque, and woke up raving when the bus entered Trinidad. The driver radioed for help. Dispatch told him to clear her aisle, belt her to her seat, and head north to Denver. Officers would be standing by.

By the time Doreen reached our floor, she was still paranoid, but the intramuscular haloperidol and lorazepam given to her in the Emergency Department had filed down the ragged edges of her agitation. She told us she had fled New Mexico to escape "vampire dealers selling me poisoned shards." She disclosed a history of schizophrenia and meth use but could not explain which came first. The medical literature provided guidance on each problem, but when it came to someone with both problems, the literature offered none of the high-level evidence we are supposed to rely upon. We were left with our own judgment. She had been calmed by an initial dose of haloperidol, so we prescribed it to treat her symptoms. She became less paranoid, but was that because of the haloperidol or because the meth was dissipating from her body? We could not say, but either way, we knew what the next step should be.

Whether her meth use came before or after she developed a psychotic disorder, it was surely one of the obstacles to health that Hildegard would have pruned away. So we asked Doreen if she was ready to quit meth. Since our unit is a teaching service, modeled after Osler's own, I let the resident make the first attempt at helping Doreen quit. He ran through a list of problems meth can cause. Anxiety. Confusion. Insomnia. Kidney damage. Lung disease. Memory deficits. Mood swings. Strokes. Tooth decay. Then he paused.

"Can you see, Doreen, why you should stop using meth? It will affect every part of your body, even your teeth."

"No, I've never had any problem with my teeth. None of my friends have problems with their teeth. They all use meth. One of my friends, she gets up in the morning, uses a little meth, gets groceries, does her prostitution thing, comes home, and makes dinner. She does fine. I do fine. Fine. Meth just helps you git. Sure, sometimes you get loopy. I mean, sometimes, I have to hide behind the dresser to keep calm. I stay there a few days. It's okay. I get hungry? My husband will chuck a burrito over the dresser. No problemo. I'm ready to head on out, get back on the bus and head for Sweetgrass, Montana."

"What's in Sweetgrass?"

"End of the highway. Sweet grass. Get it? End of the road. Where all the grass is sweet. Suweeeet." She laughed and bared her teeth. Some discoloration, poorly aligned, but intact.

She had been on the unit for a couple of days and had not acted out. She took the meds we offered her, reported feeling fit, and asked to leave. She was not ready to quit meth, but she was an adult. She forced the question: Was she ready to be discharged? Doreen was a sixty-two-year-old woman with little money, a psychotic disorder, a meth habit, and a history of disruption on the bus. For her to get back on the bus, and ride to the road's end in Sweetgrass, she would need a bus ticket from the hospital and a physician's note saying she was safe to ride. A note I would have to write.

I wanted Doreen, and everyone on the bus she boarded, to be safe, but there was no class in medical school or residency that taught us how to determine whether or when someone was safe to ride a bus. The question was critical, but there is no evidence-based answer to it, no computerized algorithm to follow.

Instead I thought of a maxim, oddly appropriate to this exact situation, that one of my senior physicians had shared with his medical students. When students asked him how they would know if a patient was ready to leave the psychiatric hospital, he told them, "If they would spook the riders on a bus, keep them overnight." We kept Doreen.

• • •

If you read medical journals and op-ed pages, you might think that prudential judgment has been banished from medical practice. Today's maxims are business maxims, such as "automation with a human touch." The traditional model of the physician as an artisan who learns how to make wise choices from master physicians is out of fashion with healthcare's technological and policy elite. The irony is that it has fallen out of fashion at the exact moment that the concept of craft is otherwise embraced. Brewers, butchers, and cheesemakers celebrate craftsmanship. They emphasize that their beer or beef or cheese was prepared according to recipes perfected over generations.

Such claims can be an affectation. Over the past decade, the meaning of foodies' favored adjectives—artisan-made, handcrafted, local, organic, and small-batch—has been exhausted by overuse. Reclaiming them for medicine seems passé. And absurd. I enjoy Trappist beer brewed the way a monastery has been brewing it for centuries, but I do not want to prescribe the medicines Hildegard of Bingen compounded in her abbey. If I fall ill, I do not want fennel seeds from a garden, but studied and standardized doses of medication and safe anesthesia. And yet, I would still want a physician who could see a patient as well as Hildegard did.

In medical school, I discovered a small book that taught me what it means to see a patient well. In *Les yeux de la foi* (The eyes of faith), the philosopher Pierre Rousselot discussed a technical philosophical question about how Aquinas understood intelligence.[1] To make the question less technical, Rousselot offered an analogy. Two detectives are dispatched to a crime scene. Upon arrival, they inspect the scene together and notice the same detail. The first detective sees the detail as a clue and solves the crime. The second detective notes the detail but makes nothing of it. While the two detectives had observed the same detail, only the former was able to make use of it.

Why could the first detective solve the crime while the second detective could not? Was the first detective simply more knowledgeable or experienced?

Rousselot insisted otherwise. He said the difference between the two detectives was that the first detective used his knowledge as a way of seeing. He saw the crime scene with his knowledge of the law, and a detail was known as a clue, allowing him to solve the crime. Rousselot wrote that the crucial difference was whether knowledge was employed as a vision: the vision of the first detective joined the proof (the clue) and what was proved (the law).

I thought of the physicians I knew and the ways they were like Rousselot's detectives. When the wise physician and unwise physician surveyed the same patient, the wise physician left the bedside with a diagnosis, whereas the unwise physician left the bedside as confused as when he or she arrived. Just as the first detective saw with the eyes of the law, the wise physician saw with the eyes of medicine.

Rousselot believed that we gained this vision by developing virtuous habits. When we engaged in the practices of the wise detective, he wrote, these practices became habits, and we eventually became wise detectives. In this formulation, a person could not learn such habits in a classroom or textbook, but only through practical knowledge. Rousselot's argument implied that medicine is called a "practice" for a reason. We learn the virtues and habits of a good physician by repeatedly performing the practices of a good physician. For the good physician, diagnosis occurs as a flash of simultaneous perception and judgment. Wise physicians can quickly resolve ambiguous problems into precise diagnoses and prescriptions.

Rousselot's account is a version of an ancient argument popularized by Aristotle. For Aristotle, we gradually achieve excellence by behaving excellently. We become just by behaving justly. We become courageous by behaving courageously. We become good physicians by performing the tasks that good physicians perform. It sounds circular. In the *Nicomachean Ethics*, Aristotle wrote both that "virtue is the result of habit" and that the virtuous "are completed by habit."[2]

Aristotle's argument has so much appeal that it has been engaged repeatedly in the centuries since he lived. Instead of focusing on the consequences of a particular action, Aristotle called attention to the qualities of the person who undertakes a particular action. He called those qualities *arete*, "virtue." "Virtue" sounds as old-fashioned as vaudeville, virginity, and the village green. So some ethicists decline to translate it, preferring the Greek *arete* to the English *virtue*. They have a point, because *arete* has resonances beyond virtue. Translators of the *Nicomachean Ethics* define it as "the excellence of a specific type of thing, animate or inanimate, that marks the peak of that thing and permits it to perform its characteristic work or task well."[3] So to have arete is really more to *be* arete, to have developed excellent habits so thoroughly that you consistently perform them over time: these habits become who you are, your character. From a virtue ethics perspective, becoming an excellent physician is less about passing examinations that assess a minimum level of competency than about pursuing the ideal of being a good physician. The work is accretive and incremental. Virtue ethics emphasizes the everyday conduct that leads to a good character. In virtue ethics, you have to be virtuous before you can achieve an evidence-based outcome or follow a checklist.

That is why virtue ethics focuses more on developing practitioners than on developing rules. A virtuous person will have developed habits that will allow him or her to achieve excellence in multiple settings. The person who learns the virtuous habits of a good physician while training in Addis Ababa should also be able to practice medicine in Amarillo, even though the technical skills required in the two settings may be distinct. Instead of developing standard work or benchmarks, virtue ethics develops people. In virtue ethics, you recognize the distinctive nature of each person by accounting for his or her particular constellation of habits. You acknowledge the relationship between habits and feelings. Finally, virtue ethics explains why a person *is* a physician rather than simply employed as a physician. Being a physician, including the social aspect of the role, both depends upon and shapes a physician's character.

The loss of our ability to account for these aspects of a physician and his or her work is part of what the older physicians are mourning when they lament what is happening to the field of medicine. Many mourn the loss of an era when physicians had more wealth and cultural privilege. (My grandmother, who lives in Amarillo, once, unbidden, took me on a drive through our hometown to show me the expensive homes of her physicians. General internists had aboveground pools, cardiologists had in-ground pools, and vascular surgeons had pool houses.) But some mourn the era when being a physician was more than a job, when it was a calling or vocation that marked a person's very character. Medical practice, they say, focused on pursuing excellence in service of an ill person, not pursuing outcomes. Outcomes and rules change all the time. New executives come to the hospital, and they prefer a different business theory. They distribute new T-shirts with new slogans. Or new regulators decide that different rules or outcomes will measure success. So when I graduated from residency, the advice a favorite teacher gave me—"Know your metrics. Rent for the first year."—was good advice for the times, advice which reflected the shifting commitments of the hospital.

• • •

The demands of the hospital, like a solvent, reveal a physician's problems even in the early days of training.

When a student at the University of Colorado fails multiple clerkships, violates the honor code, or otherwise earns a certain level of unwelcome attention from the medical school, we assemble a "success team." The team usually consists of a couple of representatives from the dean's office, physicians who specialize in academic remediation, and me. My formal reason for being there is to determine whether a student's failure has a psychiatric component.

We speak with the medical student about our concerns and considerations, but what we are really telling the student is that we doubt his or her ability to eventually practice medicine. Our implicit job is often to introduce the idea that the student will never have a career in medicine unless he or she is able to make changes he or she has, so far, been unable to make. This comes as a blow to most students, who, like their classmates, applied to medical school by writing essays about how much they liked science and helping people, and began training, usually on borrowed money, with the promise of a profession.

Any student who is smart enough to pass the exams, and stubborn enough to endure them, can get through the first two years and advance up Osler's ladder. But while hospitals like smart physicians, what they need even more are industrious and responsible physicians. So as clinical training begins, the assessments change. There are still examinations, but they make up an ever-smaller portion of students' grades. Most of a student's assessment is based on his or her ability to behave like a physician. Does the student exhibit fortitude and self-discipline, the characteristics of a physician? The assessments concern whether the student can be trusted by peers and patients.

Some students feel disoriented by the shift in assessments. A few years ago, I worked with a student who lied about patient information and claimed that he had missed rounds to care for a dying relative. His excuses were suspect and when investigated found to be threadbare fabrications. When confronted in the dean's office, he was defensive. He named his above-average exam scores and lack of interest in a particular rotation as reasons we should ignore his errors. As I listened to the student, I remembered Dr. Rogers's admonition at the white coat ceremony: "Never forget that the worst stains spill from your own character: from neglect, impatience, or greed." In attending to his intellect, the student had neglected his character.

When I think of my own errors in the hospital, Dr. Rogers's warning also pertains: my errors more often issue from my stained character than from my lack of technical skill. On my bad days, I make judgments that serve my interests rather than the interests of my patients. I answer pages slowly. When I do return calls, I offer yet another medication over the phone instead of sitting with a distressed patient.

What is difficult for medical trainees to realize is that these kinds of failings become less tolerated the farther they advance. In his classic *Forgive and Remember: Managing Medical Failure*, the sociologist Charles L. Bosk described his eighteen months following a surgical service at a teaching hospital, where he found that different kinds of errors were treated differently. He wrote that supervising physicians "tend to be tolerant and forgiving of technical error and intolerant and unforgiving of moral error. This pattern of response shows us how moral competence acts as the organizing principle."[4] Surgeons, Bosk wrote, forgave technical errors as a way to signal membership within the community of surgeons. This explains why Chapel Hill's surgeons handed out owl pins for removing healthy appendixes, while stringently punishing moral errors. These were the errors that could not be countenanced, the kinds of errors that could get a student dismissed from a training program. Or assigned to a success team.

What Bosk discovered as a sociologist is what physicians in training come to realize gradually. During the preclinical years, students believe they are studying science. Then they realize that they are not testing hypotheses but learning to apply scientific knowledge.

During the clinical years, students believe they are receiving a technical education—how to start a central line, how to alter vent settings, how to titrate a medicine. Then they recognize that they are actually being given a moral education: although many can learn technical skills, what makes a physician is the desire to use these skills well for another person, to be sure the central line is in the right place, the vent settings are correct, and the right medications are administered even when one is exhausted and irritable, and to take responsibility for any errors that occur. Students find this realization confusing because it is not why they were selected. When they applied to medical school, they knew good-hearted peers who were rejected out of hand. Medical school admission is offered not to the virtuous but to applicants with the right scores from the right schools. Then in their clinical training, they are evaluated on their character. By the time they apply to residency, they are being graded on a moral curve. Grades and intelligence still matter, but good people who are less smart are often selected for coveted spots.

There is a sense to this. In a study of medical students, trainees, and attending physicians who required remedial work at the University of Colorado, Jeanette Guerrasio and her colleagues found that professionalism deficits occurred more frequently as a physician advanced in his or her training. They also found that professionalism deficits were the best predictors that a student would end up on probation during clinical work, a finding confirmed by many other studies.[5]

So when I am involved in a medical student's success team, I listen for signs of mental illness, but what I worry about are character traits. In psychiatry, the so-called five-factor model enumerates five traits—agreeableness, conscientiousness, extraversion, neuroticism, and openness—that can be used to describe a person's character. These traits are stable over time, and the presence of a single trait—conscientiousness—is as consistent a predictor of academic success as intelligence is.[6] What I am listening for is often less about mental illness and more about whether or not a student is conscientious.

We do the same when a residency faculty meets to discuss which medical students to select for the next class of residents. The faculty values intelligence, but we require virtues like conscientiousness. So as we meet applicants, we grade them on whether they are self-disciplined and organized, whether they are developing the habits of a conscientious physician. During the resident selection process, just as during the medical school success team meetings, it becomes clear that physicians still perceive medicine as a calling, and that we still want and select for virtuous physicians.[7]

• • •

Since we learn virtue by aspiring toward ideals, our education is a necessarily social process. We need someone to emulate, someone we aspire to become. Virtue requires at least that relationship, so virtue necessarily has a social shape, formed in relationships that foster habits and character. In the Middle Ages, guilds developed as one kind of relationship for inculcating virtues. The members of guilds controlled who could and who could not belong to their confraternity, who could practice its discipline, and who controlled its supplies.

Medicine is lousy with guilds. Every specialty has its own guild, often on regional and national levels (I belong, for instance, to the American Psychiatric Association, not the Canadian Psychiatric Association). These guilds also increasingly focus on a particular part or technique. Instead of joining the American College of Surgeons, a surgeon might join the American Society for Surgery of the Hand or the Society of Laparoendoscopic Surgeons.

Despite their proliferation, the influence of these physician guilds has decreased significantly since their mid-twentieth-century apex, when the largest physicians guild, the American Medical Association, established the rules for medical practice. In 1948, when national health insurance was nearing a reality in the United States, the AMA successfully defeated the legislation through what was, at the time, the most expensive lobbying campaign in American history. Today, despite the fact that a quarter of American physicians belong to the AMA, it lacks the influence to alter legislation of that magnitude. There are many reasons for the declining influence of guilds like the AMA, but one reason is that they act less like guilds nurturing the practical wisdom of physicians and more like trade associations defending the livelihood of physicians.

This can happen even when guilds embrace prudential judgment. In 2012, the ABIM Foundation, a nonprofit organization founded by the American Board of Internal Medicine to advance professionalism in medicine, announced an initiative called Choosing Wisely. The Choosing Wisely campaign was intended to strengthen the physician-patient relationship by discouraging the overutilization of medical services. The ABIM has the support of every major medical specialty board for this initiative, in which each of the major guilds identifies five or more ways to reduce the use of expensive and unnecessary medical interventions. But the lists do not read like the maxims of yore passed on by retiring physicians. The list written by dermatologists includes, "Don't prescribe oral antifungal therapy for suspected nail fungus without confirmation of fungal infection"; the list written by internists advises, "In patients with low pretest probability of venous thromboembolism (VTE), obtain a high-sensitive D-dimer measurement as the initial diagnostic test; don't obtain imaging studies as the initial diagnostic test"; and the list written by nephrologists cautions, "Don't place peripherally inserted central catheters (PICC) in stage III–V CKD patients without consulting nephrology."[8] The name of the Choosing Wisely campaign invokes the prudential judgment of medical maxims, but its maxims will never be turned into inspirational posters or appear on a T-shirt.

These lists are evidence-based medicine summaries, compact versions of a Cochrane review, and rough drafts for the algorithms that will appear at our workstations when medicine becomes as automated as the Cheesecake Factory's kitchens. This is by design. The ABIM requires that the maxims be evidence-based. No owl pins allowed. No wisdom either, despite the initiative's title. The goal of the initiative is not, in fact, to develop the prudential judgment of physicians.

It is, like that of the kitchen managers in the Cheesecake Factory, to reduce waste in the medical system. The initiative invokes wisdom while offering algorithms. Wisdom is a quality that was once so central to society that the Greeks and Romans personified it as a divinity. Now we use it as a decoration for our formulas about the efficient and effective control of a population.

Even worse, we physicians use guilds and language about wisdom to defend our livelihoods. So when Nancy Morden and her colleagues analyzed the Choosing Wisely lists, they found that guilds rarely suggested limiting the use of their most remunerative procedures, and they often named the procedures performed by other guilds as the ones that were wasteful and unnecessary and should be discouraged.[9] We invoke wisdom, but do not practice it. We are ironic, ersatz Kraftwerkers playing at wisdom in industrial settings.

And yet virtue haunts medicine. You hear it in the medical maxims favored by the retiring physicians. You even hear it when physicians try to leave talk of virtue behind. When a group of physicians recently reviewed the various definitions of what it means for a physician to behave professionally, they found that "all expositions of professionalism, whether from professional organizations, accrediting bodies, or individual points of view, essentially devolve into descriptions of a virtuous person as physician, as well as the ways in which a virtuous physician acts."[10] We still want virtuous physicians, but we do not actively develop them, and our guilds no longer emphasize medicine as a craft learned over time in a community of wise physicians. But we still need to call on this kind of wisdom, as I realized when trying to figure out when to discharge Doreen. Thinking about the senior physician's maxim, we kept Doreen for a few more days, longer than the national standards advised or her insurer paid for, and her thinking cleared. She safely rode the bus home to a New Mexico treatment facility, wearing a T-shirt we gave her, a T-shirt without a consultant's slogan.

eleven

IMPATIENT ATTENDING

A few years into my first faculty job as an attending psychiatrist, where I saw patients and taught trainees, I was asked to direct the unit. I agreed, and the hospital printed a batch of business cards. They listed my name and my new title: "Director of Impatient Psychiatry." I passed them out for a couple years until a friend pointed out the typo. We agreed that it was fitting. Like most physicians, I like telling people what to do instead of asking if and how I can help them. Exercise more. Stop smoking. Drink less. Don't be depressed. It is a finger-wagging form of magical thinking: physician speaks, patient changes. It is never that simple, but I behave as though it is when I meet patients like Veronica.

Veronica, a twenty-nine-year-old woman who could not stop retching, came into the Emergency Department with her arms clenched over her stomach. When the urge to vomit overcame her, she released her hands so she could tightly grip the sides of a waste bin, as though she were holding on to the rails of a rolling ship. The pills she vomited into the waste bin and onto her hospital gown and the floor smelled of the antifreeze she had used to wash them down.

Once admitted to the hospital, a patient like Veronica will come my way sooner or later. No one drinks antifreeze for its health benefits. So unless you can convince the emergency physicians that it was a remarkable accident, you will be admitted to the psych service either immediately or after the internists have cleaned you out with intravenous fluids and serial blood draws. The internists declined to admit her, so Veronica was routed directly to psychiatry.

When she arrived on the unit, she told us, "I can go home. It was a mistake." I asked if she knew that this mistake could have killed her. She looked away and softly said, "I hoped so." We sat in silence. After a minute, she said, "I wanted to die."

"Do you still want to die?"

"No. Maybe. I don't know. Yes."

She told us that the previous night she had drunk eight beers, ingested some of the pills in her cousin's medicine cabinet, and fallen asleep hoping for death. When she awoke the next morning, disappointed by her failure even to kill herself, she smoked a bowl of cannabis sativa and drank the Prestone she found in her cousin's garage. Two separate attempts at suicide in twelve hours indicates a determined decision, not a sour moment.

Veronica admitted that she had been feeling depressed for three weeks. During that time, she ate less than usual, had trouble getting to sleep, felt tired most days, and lost interest in her favorite television shows. Veronica, in the technical phrase favored by gymnastic judges and contemporary psychiatrists, "met criteria" for major depressive disorder.

The evidence-based treatment algorithms for depression call for talk therapy and the judicious use of antidepressants. Both are beneficial, but they work best if their recipient is interested in changing. So when I talk with somebody about being depressed, I like to start by asking the person what changes he or she can make. When I asked Veronica, she said, "I don't know," while avoiding my gaze.

This inability to identify potential changes is a common response, even for a person who has been hospitalized for drinking antifreeze. As I was thinking about how to convince her that she had other options, the psychiatric intern broke in.

"You need to drink less, stop smoking pot, get a job, and exercise. You could run a marathon. I run marathons, and it will really help your mood to run a marathon."

Veronica stared at the intern as if she were a visitor from outer space, or at least another zip code, a more prosperous place where those choices were sanctioned and even expected. I asked, "Does that sound a little overwhelming?"

"Uh, yes."

"Can we try again?"

"Sure."

So we tried again, this time asking Veronica about her life. Whom do you live with? How do you spend your days? What do you like and dislike about yourself? As she started talking, her mood brightened, and she had ideas. She told us she wanted to move out of the house she shared with her husband because when he drank, he hit her. She thought she might take her son with her and stay at her father's house. When I asked, "When was the last time you felt hopeful about the future?" she told me it had been years.

We meet people like Veronica all the time. Discouraged, demoralized, and often depressed. They know their life is a mess. They seek help. A physician gives them a pill or tells them to run a marathon. They nod, and they return to their usual patterns or, even more unfortunately, they follow the advice and it makes things worse.

The latter was true for Veronica. Six months before we met, she visited an Emergency Department complaining of headaches. The emergency physician examined her, ordered a head CT, read the results, and sent her home with Vicodin. She took the Vicodin for a couple of weeks but hated that it made her feel foggy and bloated. A friend recommended that she ditch the pills for a natural treatment. Veronica visited her friend's marijuana physician—her friend received a free eighth of an ounce for the referral—and told the physician she had pain. Physicians in Colorado can recommend marijuana for just about anything, but most of the time they recommend it for the nonspecific diagnosis of "severe pain."[1] Veronica said the marijuana physician never asked where she experienced pain or why. He never examined her, just pulled out two forms, a permission slip to join our state's medical marijuana registry and a preprinted bill for services rendered.

While the marijuana physician filled out the forms, he asked Veronica if she had tried marijuana before. She nodded. He signed the forms and suggested she purchase an eighth of sativa next door.

When we met Veronica, we could see from her chart that she had tried marijuana before, but we needed details. She told us she first smoked at age eighteen. By the time she was twenty-three, she was smoking two or three joints a day. After about six months of this, she became despondent. While high one night, she attempted suicide by swallowing a bottle of acetaminophen. When she woke up, a plastic tube filled her trachea, an intravenous line coursed into her antecubital fossa, and a forest of IV poles and monitors surrounded her hospital bed. Over the next week, the forest thinned out, and Veronica stabilized. She was sent home at the end of the week with a referral to the local mental health center and a stack of bills she could not pay. The emergency physician had not been an employee of the hospital but a contractor who did not accept her insurance. She had bills from him, from the hospital, and from several physicians who consulted on her care while she lay unconscious. Unpaid bills were her souvenirs of these medical encounters. With more bills to pay, she had more worries, so she smoked more joints because "marijuana still relaxed me and made me less worried." It worked for a bit, but when she found work as a massage therapist, the marijuana made her too lethargic to work. She gradually stopped using it during the work week. She felt more energetic, and she eventually stopped using all together. She told us, "I kind of grew out of it."

When headaches brought her to the marijuana physician, she had not been using any marijuana at all, but at his advice she started smoking daily. The physician had, after all, recommended it. By the time we met, she had been smoking twice daily for three weeks but was still feeling some pain.

Neither the Emergency Department physician nor the marijuana physician had bothered to figure out why Veronica's head hurt in the first place. We asked. She said it had been hurting ever since her husband hit her. She told us that when she thought of him, "I carry this copper taste of fear in my mouth that he will hit me again."

There were a number of reasons for Veronica to be depressed. She told us what they were when we asked in the right way.

• • •

I sometimes ask medical students and residents to imagine walking into a bar. They see an attractive stranger and want to make the person's acquaintance. I ask how they would approach the stranger. Someone volunteers that one might use a pickup line. So I ask what pickup lines they know. They offer a few, all of which sound ridiculous while we sit, sober, in a conference room.

Then we consider a more direct approach, such as simply asking the stranger for an embrace. They all agree that unless you are a famed actor, that approach is more likely to result in a deserved dismissal than an amorous encounter.

So I ask why most physicians use one of these two approaches (or a mash-up of both) when they meet strangers as patients. We step behind curtains in the emergency department, open the door into a clinic room, or stride into an operating room and begin a barrage of scripted questions.

I call this the psychiatric robot interview. You walk into the room and immediately ask, "How is your mood? Are you having thoughts of suicide or homicide? Are you seeing or hearing things?" As an introduction to a stranger, these questions give the impression that between patient interviews, your joints will be oiled, your batteries replaced, and your operating system updated.

I spend a lot of time teaching students and residents how to talk *with* people, rather than to them, because it was something I had to learn for myself. I hate to wait my turn in a conversation, and I like to take shortcuts when I think I know where the conversation is headed. As my business cards once advertised, I am impatient and do not like to ask in the right way. I, like my resident, would prefer to direct the patient, "Do this. Don't do that. Listen to me, and you will be better." But when I think about it, I realize that such commands do not make me change my own habits, and they do not work for anybody else either. "Listen to me" never works as well as "Can I show you?" We do not receive new habits; we acquire them.

I acquired my habits reluctantly, preferring to take every available shortcut, until I realized that the shortcuts left me lost.

As a medical student, I was once interviewing a young woman who was brought to the Emergency Room with chest pain. We determined that her chest pain was caused by her cocaine use, which was sufficiently extensive that she was prostituting herself to support the habit. Because she used cocaine, I assumed that she probably used other mind-altering substances as well. Instead of asking whether she did, I took the direct route, asking, "How much alcohol do you drink in a week?" She blushed and said, "Oh no, sir, I am a Baptist. I never drink alcohol."

I made embarrassing missteps like this, whether an assumption that annoyed the patient or simply an interruption to the conversation, with every patient, and rarely was the result humorous. Usually, the patient ended up withholding information that was critical to his or her care. I would misunderstand the patient's story because, as Dr. Rogers had warned years before, one my own character stains— impatience—caused me to miss seeing the person before me. The secret of the wise attending physicians was that they put a patient at ease first, so that he or she would open up to them. Not I. I was always in a hurry, eager to obtain the data I needed from the patient so I could fill out the forms I needed to complete every day.

In residency, I learned to slow down only when I trained in psychotherapy. Time is measured differently in psychotherapy, and it is recorded differently as well. In psychotherapy you maintain an alternate chart, the supervision notebook, which you keep as an aid to memory instead of documentation to support a bill. The notebook itself is not a part of the medical record, that overgrowth of transcribed dictations, scrawled notes, and billing slips. Instead, the supervision notebook is where a psychiatrist in training writes down what goes on in the therapy room. The notebook is the record of a privileged conversation, like the notes a reporter takes in a postgame locker room, but also an emotional account of how it feels to be in that room, like the diary an adolescent keeps under the bed. The notebook is the record of two people alone in a room—one person doing most of the talking, and the other doing the listening and writing.

Once a week, I left the hospital and took the notebook to my supervisor—just as I had brought my schoolwork to my parents as a child. Supervision is the peculiar psychiatric practice that developed over the past century to answer the question of how, exactly, to train someone to perform psychotherapy. Unlike surgery, which is conducted under the bright lights of an operating suite—with many assistants, students, and trainees from several disciplines gowned and scrubbed—psychotherapy, an even more invasive procedure, is conducted alone in a closed room.

The first time I closed the door to the therapy room, all I shared with my patient was fear. I wondered whether the patient would see me for the fraud I was. What I could possibly have to offer another person? Should I behave like one of the cinematic shrinks, either coolly distant or warmly overinvolved?

I tried to remember what my teachers had advised, to ask a question and then listen, listen, listen. The resulting silence lasted for less time than I imagined, because all I could think about was failure. I wanted to speak, to retreat to the familiar ground of offering advice, but we journeyed on in the silence. When the patient spoke a word or two, it was as welcome as the first sight of land. I wrote the words down in my supervision notebook. We had a destination. Then I waited again for further direction, for more words.

The words came, week after week, session after session. I started to wonder what to do with them, how to make sense of the hesitating pauses, the false starts, the frightening statements. In the meantime, I kept writing them all down.

The supervisors were practitioners who had been performing psychotherapy for decades in the community. In medical school, I did not know that these supervisors existed. They were not the teachers who earned admirers in the lecture hall or the clinicians who wowed adherents on the wards or the researchers whose peers celebrated their publications. And yet as a resident, I learned the most from David Moore, a supervisor with whom I spent an hour each week. Moore, an Episcopal priest who had left the vestry to become a psychologist, had eyebrows that drew up into points like the crown of an evergreen and white hair that fell across his forehead to form the soft, swooping part favored by southern white men of his generation. We would meet at his home, surrounded on all sides by long-leaf pines, and sit in his office, surrounded by his books, where two chairs faced each other in a clearing.

He would ask about my cases, and I would read to him from my supervision notebooks. He would listen and then ask how it felt when a particular comment was made. I learned things from him that I could never have learned on my own. As I began to understand how to make sense of what I had recorded, I also learned how to listen and what to listen for. Finally, in his company, the advice I had received all my life—*be patient, wait your turn*—settled within me. My anxiety and worry decreased as I felt less pressured to get all my questions answered. I trusted that a patient would provide the necessary guidance in time.

David Moore conducted his practice very differently from the way I conducted mine at the hospital. The clinic rooms at the hospital were impersonal, decorated with indestructible furniture and whatever magazines had migrated from the waiting room. His therapy room was adorned with books and images of his choosing. I entered each hospital room with a preprinted billing sheet, to aid me in translating a person's experiences into an ICD-9 code and our time together into a CPT code. David entered the therapy room with empty hands.

As a volunteer member of the faculty, David gave his time freely to me, seeing me weekly in exchange for little more than an annual thank-you note from the department.

Eventually, I realized that I looked forward to our conversations because while we discussed the patients I was seeing in therapy, I was learning about my own limits, about the many things I did not do well, about how I could and could not help a person. I experienced a measure of the vulnerability my patients felt with me. I started to realize that in psychiatry, you are your own instrument; you are the tool that you employ to coax a person back to health, and to successfully wield that tool, you have to learn different ways of being with a patient.

David Moore favored an attachment-based psychoanalytic theory built around mentalization, the ability of a patient to understand his or her own mental state and the mental states of other people. Other supervisors favored cognitive behavioral therapy, intensive short-term dynamic therapy, group therapy, dialectical-behavioral therapy, or some other variant. Psychiatry has an abundance of therapeutic techniques, and many of the supervisors were adherents of a particular one. They would press photocopied articles and highlighted books into my hands, encouraging me to consider the particular technique of their favorite therapist. I went home from these sessions with texts by Habib Davanaloo, John Gunderson, Marsha Linehan, and Irvin Yalom. I sat at home trying to make sense of how their various therapies worked, then tried out the different techniques with patients. If you visited me on any given week in residency, I was equally likely to be speaking in a ginned-up therapy voice, walking about in a tweed jacket, or shopping online for a psychotherapy couch. There is a company that specializes in making them.

I was confused.

When I moved to Denver a couple of years later, Joel Yager, a senior member of the Colorado faculty, directed me to a book, *Persuasion and Healing*, which dispelled my confusion. The author, the psychiatrist Jerome Frank, had spent his career studying the efficacy of different psychotherapy techniques. He found that psychotherapeutic techniques that developed from opposed accounts of why people become ill—say biomedicine, psychoanalysis, and shamanism—could achieve similar treatment outcomes. We often attribute such findings to placebo responses, but Frank instead identified common processes for a healing relationship. Frank found that all effective healing relationships were composed of three elements: a socially sanctioned healer, a demoralized sufferer who seeks relief from the healer, and a circumscribed relationship in which they meet. Within the relationship, a healer can aid a sufferer simply by identifying a particular theory and exhibiting confidence in that theory.[2] Frank found that a therapist could discuss impaired attachments, misfiring NMDA receptors, or conflicts with dead ancestors and achieve health so long as the processes he identified were present.

Frank found inspiration for his theory in the aphorism of the Stoic philosopher Epictetus—"Men are not moved by things but by the views which they take of them."[3] Most people, Frank observed, are reluctant to change. They have fallen and can no longer imagine standing up. They have experienced an event or feeling and endowed it with a pathologic meaning. When an employer did not hire you, you were unemployable. When a girl did not return your call, you were unlovable. The truth might have been that neither the job nor the girlfriend was a good fit, but once you settled on the pathologic meanings, other possible interpretations would seem impossible. These pathologic assumptions, Frank wrote, lead to demoralization, a sense of powerlessness and passivity. The only way out of this emotional slumber is to be awakened and forced to reevaluate the meaning of the event or feeling. By turning down a date with an attractive girl or declining to hire a qualified applicant, you might come to realize that the rejections you experienced when you were younger do not always reflect upon the rejected.

If you cannot come to such a realization on your own, a healer can help. A shaman might use drums and sleep deprivation to give a new meaning to the death of your infant. Twelve-step programs might use group meetings and reflective talk to help you see why you drank so much vodka that the police had to carry you away from your mother's funeral. The cognitive-behavioral therapist might use anxiety inventories and thought records to help you understand why every time you think about your ex and his new partner, you have a panic attack that streaks your shirt with sweat. Frank concluded that in each of these kinds of encounters, a healer aroused sufficient emotion in a sufferer that the patient prepared to transform the meaning of an event. Each of these therapies, despite their manifest differences, defeated demoralization by renewing a patient's hope, increasing a patient's sense of self-mastery, and reintegrating a patient into his or her community.

Reading *Persuasion and Healing*, I wondered whether, instead of measuring physicians on the basis of their ability to generate revenue or follow standardized procedures, we could measure them by their ability to help patients make changes they could not achieve on their own. Sometimes when a patient enters a hospital, physicians might need to follow an evidence-based script, and in other cases, when perhaps the patient's problem was not a medical issue at all, physicians might need to act like a gardener and get out of the way of the body's ability to renew itself. But when a patient needs to learn a new habit, he or she may need a different kind of physician. I thought about how a physician could be more like a teacher who helps a child sounding out vowels and consonants to read sentences, paragraphs, chapters, and books. The word *doctor*, in fact, comes from the Latin *docere*, "to teach."

• • •

As I finished residency, it was my experience with teachers like David Moore that made me want to teach medical students and residents. The trouble was that, apart from decades of schoolwork, my only training as a teacher came from fitfully climbing Osler's ladder, where the phrase "See One, Do One, Teach One," was still celebrated. Teaching was a variation of clinical practice, not a skill of its own. I taught that way for a few years, but when the University of Colorado announced a new program to train faculty physicians as educators, I enrolled.

The program included faculty from all over the medical center. After years of training only alongside other shrinks, I found it refreshing to learn alongside pediatric anesthesiologists, interventional radiologists, and research pharmacologists. For a year, we spent Tuesday afternoons discussing different techniques for learning and teaching. The techniques had unexpectedly humorous names that would have worked as album titles for math-rock (Maastricht History-Taking and Advice-Scoring List) or doom metal (Death Telling Evaluation) bands. The technique that caught my ear, though, was the One-Minute Preceptor Method. In the method, the teacher follows five steps: getting a student to commit to an aspect of a patient's care, asking for evidence to support the student's commitment, teaching the student general rules, reinforcing what the student did right, and finally, correcting any mistakes the student made. The teaching model, like most of the models we learned, had been evaluated using the techniques of evidence-based medicine, in clinical trials. This was evidence-based teaching.[4]

To learn the One-Minute Preceptor, I started writing out the five steps on the bottom of the list of patients I was assigned to see each day in the hospital. I wrote the list out so I could remember to use the technique with my students and residents. Each morning, I set it down like an earnest prayer that I become the kind of teacher my students deserved. After a medical student interviewed a new patient, I would look at the list and then quiz the student. What is the patient's diagnosis? What evidence supports that diagnosis? What are the general rules for that diagnosis? What did you get right in making the diagnosis? What did you get wrong in making the diagnosis? The steps were simple, but as I went over them again and again, they improved my teaching. It became a habit to engage students on what they believed and why they believed it and then to reinforce or correct their beliefs as necessary. My teaching became more efficient and effective, but also more particular to each student. I developed a better sense of where they were and where they needed to be.

Then one morning, while listening to Veronica talk about how her husband had struck her until her head throbbed and how doctors had recommended opiates and marijuana, I grew frustrated by the ways medicine often becomes a word-association game. A patient says "depression," and we give a pill. A patient says "pain," and we dispense another pill. It makes me feel like a drug dealer, selling my wares without considering whether my customer needs them. I was frustrated that we physicians had missed the cause of Veronica's pain and subsequent self-violence, frustrated enough that, as Jerome Frank would have it, I was emotionally awakened from my usual practices. My angry eyes alighted on the five questions handwritten on my census sheet. It occurred to me that most of the time we physicians tell people what to do but do not teach them how to do it. So I wondered whether the techniques I was learning as a teacher of physicians could be of use with my patients as well.

Instead of using direct approaches and canned pickup lines—the rhetorical approaches we typically use as physicians—I started speaking with Veronica in ways that encouraged her own abilities. As I did, I felt less like a dealer and more like a teacher. Now I was helping

Veronica achieve changes she could attribute to her own efforts. Instead of being in charge of "fixing" the broken parts of Veronica, my responsibility shifted to helping her renew her hope in her ability to effect change, develop mastery over her health, and reinterpret her personal experiences.

A couple of years ago, students of Jerome Frank revisited *Persuasion and Healing*. They reviewed his conclusions and updated them with additional findings. They observed that when a patient like Veronica makes a change that she can claim as her own, it is more enduring than when she attributes it to an external source, like a medication. Frank's students found that self-efficacy, the belief that we can accomplish a given task, is a critical predictor of health. In multiple placebo-controlled psychotherapy trials (the kind Cochrane liked), Frank's students found that patients who believed in their own efficacy had better outcomes, whether they received active psychotherapy or a placebo. Behavioral changes that a patient claimed for himself or herself were more enduring than those they attributed to a physician, a medication, or a surgery.[5]

If Frank and his students are right, the first step any physician can take in helping a patient toward health is to form a therapeutic alliance with that patient. Instead of trying out the pickup line, approach the stranger at the bar with openness, and try to get to know who he or she is. A therapeutic alliance, the metaphorical dance between a patient and physician, is a relationship in which patient and physician mutually commit to the patient's well-being. This alliance is established when a patient identifies treatment goals and the physician allies with the patient in pursuit of those goals. In shrink talk, you form an alliance between yourself and your patient to mobilize healing forces within your patient by psychological means. Your ability to form these alliances profoundly influences the efficacy of your work for the patient. It also improves your satisfaction with being a physician.

Frontline physicians are increasingly exhibiting signs of burnout. In large surveys, physicians typically exhibit more signs of burnout and depression than other professionals.[6] Physicians are more likely to commit suicide than other professionals, or than the general population.[7] This might be in part because physicians feel fully responsible for too much. We feel that we have to fix what is broken, even when it cannot be fixed, even if it is not ours to fix. What if physicians were not held responsible for broken parts, but charged with renewing patients' hopes in their ability to effect change, develop mastery over their health, and reinterpret their personal experiences?

While I admire the analogy of the physician as gardener, I worry that it still assumes our control of the natural world and therefore a physician's control of the body. When I think of the physician as a teacher, I feel less dominion over the bodies of the people I meet as patients.

One morning, I found that I no longer needed to write out the steps of the One-Minute Preceptor. I had internalized them. It had become a habit to engage students and patients on what they believed and why they believed it, and then to reinforce or correct their own habits as necessary. I stopped writing out the list.

One way to renew medicine is for physicians to consider seriously how people learn and make changes in their life. If we do so, physicians like me will have to give up our roles as directors of impatience and become teachers.

It is 5:30 in the morning, and my right hand is bleeding again. I rotated a barbell knurl too fast and unhinged the epidermis from a week-old callus that had mushroomed over the base of my fifth metacarpal, and the blood-covered callus is now attached to the knurl. I stare dully at the blood and proceed on my rounds. I have six to go.

Bleeding calluses of the hand are an unusual occurrence for any physician, but especially a shrink. We develop backaches from sitting too much, sore wrists from writing too much, and headaches from hearing too much. We rarely bleed. We rarely have calluses. Our hands are usually used only for handshakes—when we fear our patients, not even for those. Lately, though, my hands have been as rough as unsettled earth, with peeling calluses on the palmar skin at the base of each metacarpal bone. It is my own fault. I joined what some call an exercise cult. I took up CrossFit.

A year into the regimen, my brother-in-law told me a joke.

"How do you know when someone does CrossFit?"

"I don't know. How?"

"They won't stop telling you about it."

CrossFit adherents have earned that reputation. We proselytize. Adherents want to tell you about the Paleo diet that many swear by, which purports to approximate the diet of our Paleolithic forebears, and they shun apostates who eat the forbidden legumes or drink the verboten milk. Some celebrate a season of fasting, the Whole Life Challenge, in which adherents advance by being more abstemious than their peers. They move through a series of constantly shifting positions, like Catholics who kneel, stand, and kneel again during a mass. They have their own language, a blizzard of acronyms and eponyms that indicate how adherents should move their bodies through those positions. They celebrate their own brand of saints' days, memorializing servicemen and servicewomen killed in combat with specific workouts that bear their names. Holleyman. Murph. Severin. Members meet in sacred spaces—neglected warehouses and service stations emptied of all adornment and furniture except those essential to their rites—which adherents call "boxes." CrossFit has it own garments, calf-high socks and technical T-shirts printed with aggro slogans and garish skulls and avenging angels that are worn by the engineers, lawyers, and physicians pursuing exercise just rigorous enough that they must purchase a special instrument to file down the calluses which disrupt their once-smooth hands.

• • •

The nurses on the psych ward were the first to tell me about Cross-Fit. Psych nurses can be salty. They spend their days stationed in a landlocked version of the medieval ship of fools, supervising an unruly collection of people shunned by society. The quarters are tight, because space is monetized in contemporary hospitals, and to the extent the unit resembles a ship, it often feels like a submarine that has been at sea too long. When we have a group of especially agitated or assaultive patients, the air becomes stale and the mood tense. We spend day after day deep in the implacable currents of madness.

Joshua spends more days in the deep than most people. In a good year, he will be admitted only once. In a bad year, quarterly. Lately, he has been stitching bad years together. Each is a variation on the same theme. His meds stop working, or he stops taking his meds. He feels good for a few days, then the pharmacokinetics collapse underneath him. His thoughts begin to race, his words to clang, and he starts adding phrases to songs, as when I heard him shout-singing, "We're gonna rock down to Electric Avenue, and then Lord Jesus will take us higher!" In the febrile moments of his mania, Joshua preaches constantly for the rapturous return of Jesus. By the time Joshua tears the clothes off his massive frame and struts naked down the Electric Avenue of his mind, he has been kicked out of another group home, and the list of places where he can live has been diminished by one, so he has to spend more days at sea in our unit, waiting to be accepted by another supervised home.

Arriving on the unit one morning, I checked in with the nurses at their station.

"How's Joshua?"

"Oh he's good. CrossFit this morning."

"What's CrossFit?"

"Oh, you know."

"No."

"Doc, he's wearing himself out by pleasuring himself."

At that point, "CrossFit" was just a new nursing euphemism to me. There are many, and like the slang of eleven-year-old boys, most relate to bodily functions. I approached Joshua's room carefully and knocked. No answer. I heard murmuring and carefully opened the door. Joshua was naked on the floor, his backside to me, his lips pressed against the return grill of the ductwork in his room. He was whispering, "Eunuch, eunuch, eunuch for the kingdom. Eunuch, unicorn, unicorn, horn, just born." I could not see his hands; whether Joshua's CrossFit session was over or ongoing, this was an occasion where I feared a handshake.

The next time I heard about CrossFit was when the cultural trend crested into my neighborhood. A few years ago, a CrossFit adherent named Neil Allman bought a modest home catty-corner to an empty gas station, its pumps long exhausted and the twin blades of its high-bay fluorescents dim on the light pole out front. He leased the gas station, replaced the fluorescent bulbs, repaired the toilet and sink, and patched a few of the holes in the walls. He removed the automobile repair bays to accommodate steel pull-up rigs and attached ropes to the ceiling so athletes could clamber up them. He covered the oil-stained concrete floor with tiles of interlocking rubber. Neil transformed the wrecked station into a CrossFit box, and within a few months, the sweat of dozens of neighborhood athletes had dripped upon the floor.

I biked by one evening and saw Neil, a blond twenty-something Übermensch, shouting instructions at a group of thirty-somethings who looked as exuberant, if more sweat-stained, as my siblings and I did while climbing over tires in our grandfather's tire shop. I stopped for a moment to watch. Every minute, a digital clock that looked like an overgrown pager would beep and they would make a rotation, from repeatedly striking a tractor tire with a sledgehammer to flipping those tractor tires across the cracked pavement to carrying weighted plates from one side of the parking lot to other and then back again. I biked past them to the gelato shop down the block, another cultural trend that had arrived in the neighborhood, but one that delivered known pleasures.

The next morning, I woke up before dawn and drove over to the hospital gym, a mirror-paneled room filled with treadmills and Cybex machines facing televisions broadcasting the overnight events from our wars. Several physicians were already strapped into the machines, earbuds in; we nodded hellos. I worked the pedals on the elliptical machine for forty-five minutes while reading medical journal articles. After completing that morning's physical penance, I shaved, showered, and dressed.

I made rounds at the hospital. I saw patients. I taught residents and students. I used the One-Minute Preceptor to ask patients and students what they believed and why they believed it, and how they could change their beliefs. As I was giving them my feedback, a resident looked shocked that I was criticizing her performance so directly. As I noticed her expression, I recalled seeing Neil outside his box, giving constant, pointed, public feedback. Instead of being discouraged, his athletes had cheered one another on as they flipped tires, swung sledgehammers, and carried weights across the wrecked surface of a parking lot. If I were looking for a way to get somebody to do something he or she would not do without prompting, it occurred to me that Neil might be able to teach me how.

I gave up on the elliptical machines.

• • •

Neil told me to come by the box for a test. When I arrived, the box was quiet. One of Neil's fellow coaches, a preposterously fit woman named Emily Schromm, was waiting for me. She asked my name and administered the test. CrossFitters call it "Baseline." Row a half-kilometer (a third of a mile) on a rowing machine, then complete forty squats, thirty sit-ups, twenty push-ups, and ten pull-ups as quickly as you can. The workout is simple but not easy. I started off quickly, before becoming winded on the push-ups and breaking the exercise into smaller sets. I did the last five pull-ups one at a time. The whole cycle took me six minutes, almost forty minutes less time than I was spending on the elliptical machine, but when I finished, I felt far more spent. Ten pull-ups was something I could not do on my own.

As physicians traverse our training, we are encouraged to focus on the activities we can do with the greatest efficiency and effectiveness. If you are a surgeon, you are encouraged to identify those procedures that you perform most successfully and stick to them. If you are an internist, you are encouraged to identify the illnesses that you treat most effectively and specialize in them. You learn the practice guidelines, the billing codes, and the quality metrics for your illnesses and confine your expertise to those areas. After a decade of having every weakness identified and explored in medical training, you find yourself, as an attending physician, playing to your strengths.

As Osler promised, seeing much had taught me what needed to be done in almost every situation that occurred on my floor, and I knew how to teach other people to do the same. After completing the Teaching Scholars Program, I was giving more feedback to students and trainees. I asked for feedback from them, but they rarely spoke as directly as I did. As I pointed out the weaknesses of my students and trainees, I started to feel cruel. I have many weaknesses and failings in need of remediation, but since I have been doing the same job every day for half a decade, they are less visible. I wanted to know again what it felt like to receive direct feedback while learning something that did not come naturally.

• • •

"Hang from the bar. Contract your shoulders. Core tight. Legs together. Pull from the hips. Push from the hips. Pull your chin over the bar."

It is five in the morning. Neil is teaching me how to perform the ten pull-ups in a row that I could not do during the baseline test. I am one of six or seven adherents awake on a frozen fall morning, and Neil is leading us through a series of exercises. We stretch, work on a skill, and then perform a combination of skills at full speed. As Neil works on the skill with me, the other athletes walk over to a bucket of gym chalk, rub a nugget of magnesium carbonate across their palms, leap to the bar, work through five, ten, fifteen, twenty pull-ups at a time, and then vault off the bar to begin the next movement. Pull-ups are a warm-up for them.

Pull-ups are a painful reminder for me. In my junior-high gym classes, boys were ranked by the number of pull-ups we could perform. I remember hanging inertly from the bar, unable to muster the force sufficient to bring my chin over the bar and thus raise me from the ranks of the athletically inadequate. Gym coaches would yell encouragement at us—"You can do it! Just do it!"—but they never taught us how to do it. Many of those coaches looked as though they had not performed a pull-up in decades. I remember looking at them with a skeptical glance, wanting to say, "I cannot *just do this*. Neither can you, you sadist."

It was because I was starting to get those kinds of looks from my own students that I found myself hanging, once again, from the bottom of a pull-up bar. Neil climbed onto the pull-up rig next to me and broke down the movement into steps. With each step, he corrected my posture, reinforced what I was doing right, and corrected my failures. When my chin did not reach over the bar, he yelled "No rep," but then taught me how to generate the extra bit of force necessary for my chin to crest the bar.

It took him two months, but I learned how to perform pull-ups. Over the next year, Neil taught me to climb a rope, to clean and jerk a loaded weightlifting bar, and to snatch kettlebells overhead—an array of movements I had believed myself incapable of. My growing ability increased my devotion. I woke up before the alarm went off, eager for that morning's challenge. As I dressed for the box, I could see how the rituals were changing my body. My clavicles were bruised from cleans, my shins were scraped from snatches, and my thighs were expanded from squats.

Physicians had specifically advised me against squatting. In high school, I ran cross-country and loved long-distance running, especially runs where we explored new terrain, but my knees did not share my enthusiasm. As we increased the distance and frequency of our runs, my knees talked back more and more pointedly. I spent half of my senior season running laps in the pool. I visited physicians and physical therapists who eventually advised me to give up running and take up the elliptical machine, where no terrain was explored, as an alternative. They told me to build up the muscles around my complaining knees, but never to lift weights and never to squat. The treatment was economical, but it taught me no new skills. I learned how to use the elliptical machine on the first day, then spent a decade on elliptical machines, going nowhere.

Neil told me the opposite: learn to squat, and then squat often, with escalating weights. He taught me to air squat without weights, then to back squat with a weighted bar balanced on my shoulders, then to front squat with the bar pressing against my clavicles, and to overhead squat with the bar held above my head. I learned to pistol, squatting on one leg while holding the other in the air before me. Of all the weightlifting movements we performed in the box, I was best at squatting, the very activity physicians had told me to avoid. After six months of squatting, my decade and a half of knee pain was over, and I resumed long-distance running. I ran my first half-marathon at a faster pace than I had run in high school, the kind of experience that makes a true believer of one.

These experiences raised questions. How many of my patients are similarly stuck in unnecessary, physician-recommended regimens? Should I, as a physician, be more like Neil, more like a kind of coach?

The first question was difficult to answer, but I decided to put the second to the test. With students and trainees, translating Neil's approach was fairly straightforward. Neil worked with each of his athletes differently, encouraging a fearful athlete to try a more advanced movement and discouraging a reckless athlete from lifting a dangerous weight. For both kinds of athletes, he would break down a movement into its constituent steps, so that they could learn one piece of the movement at a time, instead of being asked to perform the entire movement on the first day. So when students or trainees join our team, we meet on the first day and I ask for a description of a teacher or coach for whom they excelled. Together, we identify what motivates a student or trainee and how he or she learns. Watching Neil led me to break my comments into smaller steps. I take notes as a student or trainee interviews a patient. Afterward, I identify a misstep or two and discuss alternate approaches, rather than simply observing that an interview did or did not go well.

The trouble comes with translating Neil's approach to patients like Joshua.

The literal translation would be to join my patients in our unit's daily group exercise class. On occasion, a yoga instructor visits and leads the patients through poses. These sessions are well received, but the most disturbed patients frighten many yoga instructors, so we find that after a few sessions the teachers are less interested. Joshua, in fact, has seriously assaulted a staff member in the past, so lying next to him in corpse pose is a lot to ask of a volunteer yoga teacher.

More commonly, staff members lead the group exercise class. They do a few generic stretches and then insert one of two donated videotapes into what might be North America's last working combination VHS-TV machine. When the patients are a bit rowdy, the staff plays a Tai Chi videotape, in which the mulleted and mustachioed instructor over-enunciates Chinese phrases and frequently invokes "My Master" while making slow movements through the air. When the patients are more lethargic, the staff plays a Billy Blanks Tae Bo videotape, in which Blanks wears a singlet that stops below his oiled nipples and prances around a studio set thrusting his legs and hands in the air. Whenever I arrive on the unit and find the patients exercising, I always stop to watch. The videos seem to be teaching viewers less about how to make peace with embodiment or to exercise, and more about how to be a narcissist. Look directly into the camera. Speak in catchphrases. Surround yourself with smiling sycophants mimicking your moves. Endorse your own line of workout clothes.

Both videotapes allow the staff—who are, after all, punished or rewarded based on how well they document patient care, rather than on their ability to motivate patients—to catch up on charting from the comparative safety of the nursing station. And some patients love the videotapes and will happily spend a full hour with Mr. Tai Chi or Billy Blanks. But most lose interest after a few moments; like the rest of us, the patients find it harder to complete the workout if they have to supply the motivation. So I sometimes fantasize about leading patients through chest-to-bar pull-ups and double-unders and Turkish get-ups.

Then I realize that this fantasy is one in which I impersonate Neil, in which I give up on medicine in favor of becoming a literal coach, while missing the lesson he taught me about being a physician.

• • •

Among CrossFit initiates, there is a popular saying: "Your physician is a lifeguard, not a swim coach." The saying comes from a videotaped lecture by Greg Glassman, the founder of CrossFit, which adherents recirculate on social media. In the lecture, Glassman explains that physicians, like lifeguards, watch life's action from a distance, intervening only when a problem develops. If you tear your ACL, a physician will repair it, but if your knee pain can be controlled by time on the elliptical machine, earbuds in, there is no need for a physician to intervene. In contrast, Glassman claims that CrossFit coaches are like swim coaches who teach you how to move differently before a problem develops. If your knee has pain, Glassman says you need to get off the elliptical machine and learn to move differently. Glassman contrasts the passive nature of most fitness programs with the active challenges of CrossFit.[1]

Like many of Glassman's statements, this is an admixture of insight and overstatement. We need a lifeguard sometimes. Still, I take his point that we physicians ought, more often, help people improve their health the way a coach does. Neil certainly helped me.

There are no mirrors in Neil's gym, no sycophants watching you exercise, and no one charting your movements on the sideline. There is, as in most CrossFit boxes, a dry-erase whiteboard mounted to the wall, where adherents keep track of their own records. When I look at the whiteboard and compare myself to the other athletes, I feel the same sharp fear I used to feel when I looked at hospital whiteboards and saw a list of new patients. Like those lists, where the patients changed daily, no record in the box is permanent, and each athlete is forever seeking a new personal record, the ability to perform a new movement or complete the "WOD," workout of the day, "Rx," as prescribed by the coach. The pursuit of mutual betterment through personal records is central to the social structure of the box. Working together, we push one another to complete one more round. I do not want to quit when the person beside me is working her or his way through another round, even when my calluses are bleeding. Persevering side by side builds community. So does the program, which is constantly varied to identify and address individual weaknesses.

My weakness remains muscle ups, a movement that combines speed, strength, and skill. You leap up and grab hold of gymnastic rings positioned just out of standing reach. With your legs together, toes pointed out, you pull yourself up so the rings are level with your sternum, then push down on the rings down so that they are tight against your hips, and you are balancing in the air. On one level, this is just a pull-up followed by a dip, two moves you learn early in CrossFit. The difficulty lies in the skill it takes to get from a pull-up to a dip while maintaining your balance in the air. The muscle up is a movement that is usually perfected by gymnasts, not physicians, and mastering the muscle up distinguishes the skilled adherents of the box from the merely committed.

It was muscle ups that the other members were working on when I started learning pull-ups on my first day. On the day I joined, they did not ask what I did for living—it was months before someone did— but whether I could do a muscle up. When I said no, they offered encouragement rather than condemnation. In the box, what matters are the movements you can perform, the weights you can lift, and the workouts you can survive working alongside each other.

In that respect, the box resembles a religious community. What matters is your participation in the life of the community, not your life outside the box. Neil reinforced this, sending reminders about missed sessions, passing out free vegetables from his backyard garden, and organizing community dinners for holidays and good-bye parties when a member moved out of town. Like communal meals in a religious community, these meals adhered to a specific diet. There were a lot of kale chips and bacon-wrapped dates washed down with tequila shots.

Over the past few decades, there has been a growing interest in translating the work of coaches like Neil into medicine. Most of this interest is, blessedly, less literal than my fantasy of doing rope climbs and kettlebell swings with persons hospitalized with a serious mental illness.

One adaptation is a variation of psychotherapy called health coaching. As in other forms of psychotherapy, the first step is building an alliance with a patient. In most forms of psychotherapy, a patient then identifies a problem. In health coaching, a patient typically identifies an area for improvement. In traditional psychotherapy, we often help a patient discern the relationship between past events and the patient's own present condition. In health coaching, the therapist typically focuses only on present conditions. I work as a kind of health coach when I engage in motivational interviewing. Motivational interviewing, like the One-Minute Preceptor model, depends on getting someone to commit to a belief, exploring the evidence for the belief, and assessing his or her willingness to make a change.

You can engage even profoundly ill patients, like Joshua, in motivational interviewing.[2] Some days we talk about what his medications do for and to him. Some days we talk about his desire to live in an apartment of his own. Some days we talk about whether he will strut unclothed around the unit or get dressed. With motivational interviewing, you can always identify a change that someone, even a patient as visibly ill as Joshua, wants to make. The work is satisfying to me because the interaction is less about telling a patient what to do than about motivating a patient to change. When I act as coach to someone like Joshua, I accept approbation or credit only for the extent to which I am able to motivate a patient to attempt to take action. It feels more honest and bearable than full responsibility.

A growing literature of rigorous evidence, the kind Archie Cochrane feared psychiatry could never achieve, supports the efficacy of health coaching, motivational interviewing, and related techniques like cognitive behavioral therapy. Cognitive behavioral therapy can be as effective as medications for many people with mental illness. Motivational interviewing is an extraordinarily effective way to help a person overcome addiction. Health coaching improves control of chronic diseases like diabetes and hypertension.[3]

The authors of this literature are enthusiastic about the benefits of health coaching. They write that coaching is focused on health rather than illness and on patients' needs rather than physicians' skills. Coaching can be delivered by professionals with far less training than physicians: a diabetic can teach another insulin control, a former alcoholic can coax someone to sobriety, a dynamic certified nursing assistant can help a person quit smoking.

But there are limits. Many kinds of health coaches and patient navigators have, like CrossFit instructors, modest training credentials. Since much of healthcare is routine, modest training is often sufficient. When rare events disrupt the routine, though, modest training can be dangerous. In many respects, the inconsistent training of health coaches, patient navigators, and CrossFit instructors resembles medical training before Flexner's *Report*, in that the outcomes depend largely on the character of the coach, navigator, or instructor. Another problem is that for coaching to work, an individual must have some desire to be coached. Those are significant obstacles to adapting the lessons of CrossFit to patients like Joshua. Over the past few years, we have referred him to peer support groups and health coaches. They inevitably dismiss him from their practices, apologetically explaining that he is simply too ill for their services. One told me, "I know he speaks English, but it was honestly like he was speaking a foreign language when he came around." Sometimes, you need a lifeguard.

• • •

CrossFit has earned its adherents and its critics. Serious weightlifters and gymnasts complain that boxes reduce their training regimens into mere exercise. Concerned physicians and trainers worry that teaching relatively unskilled people to perform demanding weightlifting and gymnastic movements leads to injuries.[4] (Full disclosure: I have chipped a tooth and herniated my anterior tibialis muscle, but both injuries fell under the sign of Cochrane's declaration that "doctors are superfluous" and required no medical attention.) And there are concerns about inadequate training for coaches.

These criticisms have merit, and I recognize that CrossFit is a fad whose time will pass (who still Jazzercises?), but it has taught me something about what to hope for in medicine. I wonder whether it could teach others in medicine as well.

In his lectures, Glassman celebrates the ways CrossFit creates community. Glassman developed the idea of CrossFit, but has no ownership or managerial role in local boxes. Glassman wants owners to focus on their box and its athletes, so he prohibits an affiliate owner from opening multiple boxes. Each box is determinedly local, named after neighborhoods rather than cities or states, so I go to CrossFit Park Hill, not CrossFit Denver. Within the box, the owner decides on the programming, hours, and rules. The creators of CrossFit have figured out how to transform the physical health of millions while allowing someone like Neil to create a community around his box. In contrast, hospitals have been able neither to achieve the health outcomes they desire for their patients nor to maintain local control. We are turning hospitals into factories owned by large corporations, insisting that only its economies of scale can achieve consistent outcomes. The growth of CrossFit suggests that we could still engage millions of people in an activity while allowing significant local control.

Of course, there are limits to how far CrossFit's principles can be extended. Part of why it is easy for me to see how to be a coach to residents and trainees is that we are on a continuum, occupying different rungs on Osler's ladder. They began their journey with no assistance from me and are internally motivated. They want to climb the ladder. The same is true at a CrossFit box. You join only after you volunteer for it. Joshua never volunteered for his illness, and he resents his encounters with a medical system that struggles to engage him in conversation. Anyone who knows Joshua will agree that he says remarkable things, but it is difficult to know what they mean. A recent conversation went like this:

"How are you?"

"My heart is indicting a good theme."

"Why?"

"Roy Orbison is a good singer, but we don't have to do everything he says."

Joshua knows the language game of physician and patient better than anyone should. Physicians have seen him at least monthly for the past three decades. He has worked with two generations of psychiatrists and has been prescribed every fad medication around. Sometimes Joshua plays the language game of medicine with his physicians, and sometimes he chooses not to. Sometimes he is simply unable to play patient to the physician. At those times, his thoughts are racing, his ideas flying, and his non-sequiturs might as well belong to a foreign language.

At those times, I become to Joshua what my junior high coaches were to me, a person who demands that he do things he simply cannot do on his own.

Coaches can use techniques like motivational interviewing to kindle and encourage patients and students, but profound illness incapacitates self-motivation. Joshua is neither weak-spirited nor lazy. He is ill. Learning a muscle up—a task I still have not mastered after three years of thrice-weekly sessions—is challenging, but surely overcoming psychosis is a task of a very different order.

Maybe the best way to take advantage of the benefits of CrossFit is to take away the idea not of the coach but of the community of adherents. CrossFit is expensive, but I keep returning to the box, even after Neil moved away and sold the box to a new owner, Michelle Kinney. I still return every week because I am eager to learn new skills in a community that uses some of the techniques of a religious community—a purified diet, a ritualized space, a specialized language, and a communal life in which alliances develop among adherents. Perhaps medicine could use religious techniques to effect change in the lives of patients. That was the hope that first sparked my interest in medicine.

I decided to become a physician when I collected Franciszek from an Emergency Department in Chicago. At the time, I was young and angry. Franciszek was old and intoxicated.

I had seen high school drinking and college drinking—intoxicated friends acting exuberantly and stupidly. They pulled down curtains or kissed strangers or threw punches. At their worst, they looked cruel.

At his worst, Franciszek looked desolate. His poorly dyed hair had receded, leaving no shade for the bruises on his forehead. The bruises matched the hematomas on his arm, where the phlebotomists had drawn blood and the nurses had started fluids. Taped to his left cubital fossa, inside his elbow, was that day's intravenous needle, dripping saltwater and thiamine into his vein. He had fallen down drunk and woken up, again, in an Emergency Department detox bed.

When I arrived, many people were waiting to be seen. But when I told the clerk that I was here to collect Franciszek, a homeless Polish immigrant, a nurse immediately came over.

"Did you know this loser has been in my ED fifteen times in the past thirty days?"

"No, I didn't. Has he been a problem?"

"No, he's always calm, just really drunk and tearful. Pathetic."

She handed me Franciszek's medical record and pointed to the blood-alcohol levels from his admissions—314, 457, 512—levels that would have killed the college drunks I knew. While I tried to figure out the medical record's abbreviations and scribbles, she abruptly pulled back the curtains around Franciszek's borrowed bed. Franciszek lay curled up without opening his eyes, whimpering like an abused animal. She flapped on all the lights with a sweep of her left hand. With the knuckles of her right, she rubbed his chest and yelled, "Your ride is here. Ride is here. Time to go. To go. Go!"

I was the ride, a twenty-two-year-old AmeriCorps volunteer at Interfaith House, a respite center for the homeless on Chicago's West Side. The center had a deal with several hospitals: If a hospital agreed to provide follow-up care, the center would allow the hospital to discharge its homeless patients to the facility. We would house and feed them and sign them up for whatever housing, services, and jobs we could find. My job was whatever unskilled work needed doing each day. I cleaned closets, administered drug tests, and admitted new people. When the staff driver was unavailable, I drove the passenger van, taking people to the medical appointments promised them by the discharging hospitals. I got to know Chicago by figuring out where every community health clinic, dialysis center, and hospital was located.

That day, I was sent to pick up Franciszek. He had identified the center as his next of kin. No one at Interfaith House was literally related to Franciszek, but we knew him as well as anyone did. A year before, he had crashed his truck and woken up hungover in another hospital with a compound tibia fracture. He lost his commercial truck driver's license and with it his job, income, and apartment. With nowhere to go, he accepted the hospital's referral to Interfaith House. Unlike most people, who stayed less than a month before they tired of the hassles attendant on sharing a building with sixty homeless strangers, he had stayed for ten months. He got sober, healed his leg, and became a role model. He helped out with the grounds, secured a job, and met with donors to show off what the center could do. He was our success story, our family's prodigal son restored to health. The center's social workers found him a studio apartment in a nearby Polish neighborhood and furnished it with secondhand furniture. On the day he left, we held a party and served cake and punch. We celebrated ten clean months during which his reticent smile had returned and his rounded spine had straightened. It was a graduation party sponsored by his social services family.

I thought about what it would be like to have no family except for social services personnel as I collected Franciszek from the hospital. When the nurse pulled back the curtains and enveloped Franciszek in sterile light, he began thanking me. Something decent in me grasped his left hand while the nurse hectored him to sign discharge papers with his tremulous right hand. She removed his intravenous line without a word and, tasks accomplished, wheeled him out of the room. As she pushed his hospital bed, she dropped the rails as though she were opening the pen of a bum steer, and shoved him into a wheelchair. As I wheeled Franciszek toward the door, a physician said, "See you next time." I wanted to spit and mutter something indecent.

Franciszek cried as we drove down Pulaski. His lips, frosted white from dehydration, quivered. He smelled of the cheap schnapps he favored. He was ashamed, and his eyes never met mine as he attempted justifications, but his stories returned, inevitably, to the single certain fact of his life.

He drank.

Before that afternoon, I had been undecided about my future. Record-store clerk? Sportswriter? English teacher? I was confused, in the privileged way that young liberal arts graduates are often confused, by my plethora of choices. On that day, though, I was confused by Franciszek's condition and the way he was received at the hospital. I was naive, believing that nurses and physicians were supposed to serve Franciszek instead of humiliate him.

Franciszek and I returned to the center. I asked him to wait in the admissions room while I gathered the intake forms. He nodded and sat with his eyes cast down at the beige linoleum of the admission room, the room where we went through the belongings of the newly admitted, throwing out bottles of sugared rotgut, boxes of improvised crack pipes, and the bags of store-brand corn starch which could trick a hungry stomach into feeling full. The floor was pitched at an angle, causing his possessions to roll away from him, as they had for the past few years. Over those years, Franciszek had become accustomed to the invasions, the interminable waiting, and the impersonal forms of service agencies. To hasten the process, I started on the intake forms using records from his previous admission, the first of many times I would start the documentation of a patient encounter before seeing a patient. With the forms prefilled, I only had to ask Franciszek a few questions.

"Anything bothering you physically?"

"No."

"Any sense of why this happened again?"

"Alone, I am alone. I drink."

"Anyone you want me to call?"

"No."

I did not know what to say. I completed the forms. I rifled through the clear plastic bag labeled "Patient Belongings" with which the hospital had discharged Franciszek. I showed him to a bed.

I left the building, started a borrowed car, turned the stereo up, and listened to a mixtape from a friend back home. As the songs propelled me across Chicago, every good I could imagine felt undone. The ten months of Franciszek's sobriety had ended, the fruits of the staff's labor had proved short-lived, and the physicians and nurses at the local Emergency Department had revived him without welcoming him.

With my brooding thoughts, I made my way south to the Dominican priory where I was living with a group of friars and priests—some in training, some active, some retired—who sponsored the AmeriCorps program in which I was enrolled. The idea was that AmeriCorps volunteers spent their days at a local social service agency and their nights and weekends living with the Dominicans as a way of experiencing a life of service. The priory was a massive four-story brick building built during boom times for the Catholic Church, when priories bustled with young Dominicans. By the time I arrived, the long bust had begun, and there were enough free rooms to provide a private room for each volunteer.

I returned home that evening in time for vespers. A few months earlier, I had been in college, where I could return to the dorm when I chose and do what I pleased when I got there. If I had been still in college, I would have spent the evening alone with my festering resentments, but at the priory I was expected to attend vespers. The community's modest chapel was on the first floor; no one could sneak into the house without passing it. I took off my winter coat and dutifully collected a hymnal. I entered the chapel and found a seat in wooden pews that faced each other. The brothers and priests looked almost as disinclined to be there as I was. Still, we all opened our hymnals and sang, off-key, from the seventy-second psalm: "He will rescue the poor at their call, / those no one speaks for. / Those no one cares for / he hears and will save, / save their lives from violence, / lives precious in his eyes."[1] I thought of Franciszek. When he would be rescued? When would his life be saved? The hymn left me hungry for an unfulfilled promise, but at least we named that promise, and named it together.

The Dominicans, however, seemed more like grumpy bachelors than holy celibates. They followed evening vespers with plates of pot roast and potatoes, then rode the elevator up a flight to the lounge, where we sat in worn recliners, sipping cut-rate scotch and watching laugh-track sitcoms. These men had joined their lives together, but I never seriously considered paying the admission price of celibacy for their version of communal life. The prospect of fighting over the remote with thirty other men for the rest of my life was another disincentive.

The communal life I found more compelling was the life enjoyed by their sister community, the Sinsinawa Dominicans. Whereas the brothers and priests seemed similar to the other resigned middle-aged Midwestern men I knew, the nuns seemed strangely alive in the absence of men. Indeed, when I visited their motherhouse in rural Wisconsin, it seemed as though they never died. Walking along the sunlit halls, I met an octogenarian who was still teaching elementary school, a nonagenarian serving as spiritual director to the novices, and a centenarian who read to the blind. The priory smelled of menthol, but the motherhouse smelled of the sweet breads the sisters sold to support themselves. When they sang together, they sang boldly and in harmony. Afterward, they talked eagerly of their work as they sat at table. I met nuns who taught nearby and in Nicaragua, nuns who ran hospitals, and nuns who worked in hospitals as nurses or physicians.

Those women intrigued me. I had never met a nun who was also a nurse or physician, a contemporary Hildegard of Bingen. When I mentioned this to the one of the sisters, she laughed and told me nuns had been working as nurses and physicians for millennia, founding hundreds of hospitals in the United States alone. She said that when she was a teenage novice, her community sent her to medical school. She had come from a farming family and never imagined she could become a physician, but she went to medical school because her community called her to the practice. That sounded like precisely the kind of communal direction I was looking for, so I started telling her about Franciszek and the other people I met at Interfaith House. When I got to the part about singing the seventy-second psalm and longing for its promise, she asked if perhaps I should serve by becoming a physician, handed me a holy card, then moved on to her next conversation.

I never really thought of physicians as servants. As a child, the white-coated physicians I knew were kind-hearted and civic-minded, but bourgeois, professionals. They drove better cars and lived in larger houses than their neighbors. They offered a professional's service for a professional's fee. When I worked at Interfaith House, I talked daily to people discharged from Chicago's hospitals. Few spoke of being served by a physician. When I looked over the medical records sent with them from the hospitals, I saw only indecipherable codes written by numerous physicians. When I accompanied a patient on medical visits, the physicians seemed to be, like those who had treated Franciszek, curt technicians who dismissed the patient after ensuring that he or she was no longer in imminent danger. I had never met a physician whom I could describe as a servant, but this nun assumed that physicians served.

• • •

Puzzled by the nun's suggestion, I started looking for evidence of physician-servants.

She had given me a holy card, the Catholic version of a baseball card, for two saints I did not know, Cosmas and Damian. On the front, the saints were portrayed as fresh-faced boys in matching halos, red velvet robes, and green calf-length gowns. They looked as though their pious mother had dressed them up for the third-century version of the family Christmas card. The back of the card bore the caption "Physicians and Martyrs" and a prayer, written in the passive plea of the genre, that these saints would transform the bearers into "willing and loving servants."

Curious, I started looking around used bookstores for more information on these saints. Few sections of a used bookstore are as neglected as the medicine or the religion section; the books that straddle the two are invariably dusty and marked down. In that overlap, I found books whose covers included stethoscopes transmuted into religious symbols, books with heroic portraits of once-charismatic authors, and a series of pamphlets, one of which mentioned that Cosmas and Damian were acclaimed as "holy unmercenaries," or "as doctors without silver," because they would never accept payment for the medical care they provided.[2] Sounded like hagiography to me; I could not imagine physicians working without pay.

I moved on to the bioethics section, where I found a book called *Suffering Presence*, by Stanley Hauerwas. The back cover promised that it addressed key questions in bioethics. I brought it home and skipped sitcoms and scotch in favor of reading it that evening. I had never really read theology before and was engaged by its rhetorical force. Hauerwas did not engage in tedious methodological arguments, like the postmodern critical theory I labored through as an undergraduate, but sounded deep questions about illness and health. I did not register the entire argument, but I understood his claim to be the same as the nun's. It was once commonplace, he wrote, for a physician to conceive of himself or herself as a servant commissioned by a community, and he argued that this conception was still necessary. I underlined such passages as "Medicine needs the church not to supply a foundation for its moral commitments, but rather as a resource of the habits and practices necessary to sustain the care of those in pain over the long haul."[3] Hauerwas wrote that if medicine did not have the church or a community similar to one, physicians would not be able to endure being present to suffering of their patients. Without a community, physicians would be overwhelmed by that suffering and become alienated from the ill people they were supposed to serve. If a community called physicians to serve the ill, however, then they could fulfill their vocation, "to serve as a bridge between the world of the sick and the world of the healthy."[4]

Hauerwas believed physicians could be a bridge between the ill and the well, but I had seen little of that in my work with the homeless, so I wrote him a letter telling him so. He wrote back, asking me to work for him that summer. A few months later, I left Franciszek and the brothers in the priory and moved to Durham, North Carolina, to work for Stanley. When I arrived, he gave me a stack of books to read, several boxes of papers to organize, and a question.

"What do you want to be?"

"A bioethicist."

"People think bioethicists are assholes. They tell everybody what to do but don't do it themselves. You need to serve somebody. You should go to medical school."

I figured that was the closest I would ever come to a commissioning.

• • •

While waiting to start medical school, I looked for signs of physicians who worked as servants, without silver.

Stanley Hauerwas introduced me to the Catholic Worker, a loose-knit group of anarchists, pacifists, and former altar boys who operate houses of hospitality for the poor. The houses engage in various works of art, agriculture, education, medicine, prayer, and resistance in the spirit of their founder, Dorothy Day. For a year, I volunteered occasionally at House of Grace, a Catholic Worker house run by two women, one a nurse practitioner. On weeknights, she would see ill patients in a rundown row house. On the first floor, we volunteers would run a warm shower for patients who were dirty and bring a plate of food to patients who were hungry. When the nurse practitioner was ready, we would escort the waiting patients upstairs, past an indifferently displayed collection of radical posters and holy cards. One evening, I noticed the Cosmas and Damian card among their number. The tradition of the holy unmercenaries, the doctors without silver, was alive, at least in that row house.

I told myself that being unmercenary was fine for them, but too much for me. I was still a student; they were practitioners. I was accumulating student loans; they had paid theirs. Excuses, of course, but I kept looking for a more approachable way to be a physician-servant.

I lived in a commune for a year, but I grew tired of the bickering and the vegan dinners. At least the Dominicans served scotch.

I also read the books of David Hilfiker, a physician who worked for several years in a rural private practice before joining a Protestant analogue of the Catholic Worker in an impoverished neighborhood in Washington, D.C. Reading Hilfiker was bracing: he disclosed the emotional challenges of practicing medicine, of bearing full responsibility. Instead of writing about his triumphs, he wrote about his mistakes. And instead of using his mistakes as the rhetorical grounds for the need for a better laboratory test, a larger evidence base, or a quality-improvement initiative, Hilfiker understood them as a reminder of his own limits and the limits of medicine. He advised physicians to abandon their pretense of perfection. He eventually concluded that the only way to throw off the yoke of perfection was to live among the poor patients he served. He gave up his isolating bourgeois life as a private practitioner for a communal life, in which he and his family lived with the indigent ill, in order to practice medicine as a servant, and as one who could admit his mistakes and be forgiven for them.[5]

Hilfiker's honesty and service seemed both ideal and impossible to me—I was more reluctant than "willing and loving"—so I tried to approach it with an analogue. When I started medical school, I signed up as a volunteer at the school's free medical and dental clinic. It was open one night a week, and while the number of patients ranged from two to twenty people, the clinic was always well staffed with eager volunteers from the university's medical, nursing, pharmacy, physical therapy, public health, and social work schools. A student from each discipline saw every patient. A patient presenting with a straightforward complaint—a mandatory school physical, a simple urinary-tract infection—endured a three-hour exam, swarmed about by well-intentioned students. An efficiency expert could have taught us a great deal about how to run that clinic.

Although I enjoyed my time in the clinic, in hindsight, I recognize that it was far more helpful for me than for the patients. Volunteering in the clinic was a weekly reminder of why I enrolled in medical school, something I needed during days of indifferent lectures, even if it was only an abstraction of the House of Grace or Hilfiker's clinic. We did not live with our patients. We drove to the neighborhood, provided a student's version of a professional's service, and then drove home. For all our good intentions, the student clinic was another iteration of the training wards of Osler's hospitals, where the bodies of the poor and the indigent were the pathology textbooks for student practitioners. Patients received care without charge, but they did so in exchange for functioning as a textbook.

I continued searching for my version of the physician-servant, and my search led me back to Stanley Hauerwas. He convinced me to take a leave of absence from medical school to study the history of physicians as servants with him.

• • •

In my medical school, the history of medicine began with an invocation of Hippocrates and his oath, then jumped ahead to Ignaz Semelweiss and his efforts at antisepsis. The less said about the intervening centuries, the better. But Stanley wanted me to look at those intervening years.

He taught me about the initial break between Platonic and Hippocratic medicine. In Platonic medicine, a physician sought to diagnose disease as an ontological entity, a concrete fact that should be named rightly. A competent Platonic physician identified the disease the patient had. In Hippocratic medicine, a physician sought to understand an ill person by learning the beneficial and deleterious forces in his or her life, and then helped a patient as he or she sought repair. A competent Hippocratic physician understood the patient.[6]

Stanley Hauerwas showed me that even though Hippocratic physicians sought understanding, they did not seek the solidarity with the ill that servants such as Hilfiker or the Catholic Workers or the nun from the Sinsinawa Dominicans sought. To illustrate the difference, he gave me Guenter Risse's *Mending Bodies, Saving Souls: A History of Hospitals*. Risse wrote that, for Hellenistic physicians, the god Asclepius was the paradigm. In Asclepius's temples, an ill believer entered into an exchange relationship with the deity, giving gifts for health. In the clinics and hospitals of Hellenistic physicians, an ill believer likewise entered into an exchange relationship with the physician, paying a fee for the physician's services. Asclepius saw only the ill who sought him out, worshipped him, and made sacrifices in his name. So Hellenistic physicians saw only the ill who entered into the exchange relationship between patient and physician. In ancient Greece, Risse wrote, there "was no public duty toward the sick" because "illness remained a private concern."[7] If you were ill, you could receive succor from your kin or, if you had the means, enter into an exchange relationship with a physician. There was no public philanthropy for impoverished or estranged ill people.

Social welfare for the indigent became a communal responsibility, Risse wrote, only with the rise of the Jewish tradition of hospitality to the dispossessed and the Christian tradition of charity to the indigent. Jewish and Christian physicians practiced the Hellenistic medicine of their era—they did not develop a unique account of medicine, of why people fall ill, the treatments they should receive, or how they were restored to health—but were distinguished from other physicians by why they practiced medicine and for whom they practiced it.

In the Diaspora, Hellenistic Jewish physicians had a particular interest in the poor and the stranger because they belonged to a community formed by prophetic hopes for something more than fee-for-service relationships with deities. I saw this in the book of Micah, where the prophet called his hearers to approach God with virtuous behavior instead of sacrificial offerings:

With what shall I come before the LORD, and bow before God most high?
Shall I come before him with burnt offerings, with calves a year old?
Will the LORD be pleased with thousands of rams, with myriad streams
  of oil?
Shall I give my firstborn for my crime, the fruit of my body for the sin of
  my soul?
You have been told, O mortal, what is good, and what the LORD requires
  of you:
Only to do justice and to love goodness, and to walk humbly with
  your God.[8]

The people who heard and transmitted this text were called not just to be competent in exchange for a fee, but to be virtuous servants who performed works of mercy.

The Gospel of Matthew describes Jesus delivering a similar list of the works of mercy to his followers at the peak of his public ministry—"I was hungry and you gave me food, I was thirsty and you gave me drink, a stranger and you welcomed me, naked and you clothed me, ill and you cared for me, in prison and you visited me."[9] Although this list of the works of mercy would be familiar to Jewish communities as *gemilut hasadim,* the meaning of the works was altered when Jesus identified himself with the hungry, the thirsty, the stranger, the naked, the ill, and the imprisoned—the least-valued people in society. Jesus called his disciples to attend to those who are ill, poor, weak, or powerless as the way to attend to him.

In the first centuries after the death of Jesus, his followers debated to whom the text was addressed. Should the followers of Jesus serve only other followers of Jesus? Early Christians including Jerome, Augustine, John Chrysostom, and Gregory of Nyssa insisted that the followers of Jesus must serve all humanity—especially the least—and their interpretation became normative.

Jesus told his followers to see the ill as a servant would, whether they were serving food to the hungry or tending the sick. The servant's gaze was quite different from the clinical gaze that I was being trained to use in medical school, where seeing patients in terms of parts and money seemed like an updated version of sacrificial exchange offerings. I watched every day as patients entered the hospital as though it were a temple, with high hopes for what its practitioners could accomplish, and exited days or weeks later with bills they could never pay. When I asked attending physicians how much the tests and studies we were ordering would cost our patients, none could answer. One attending thought my questions signified an interest in billing, so he pulled me aside and showed me documentation tips to optimize my future salary. You needed at least three items in the review of systems. You needed specific diagnoses. You needed to document your time, because you were paid for it.

I appreciated being taught the mechanics of the exchange offering, but I wanted to know what a place shaped by the works of mercy looked like, a place were you saw patients like a servant.

Stanley Hauerwas taught me that public hospitals were built to perform the works of mercy. The first public hospital was built by Basil of Caesarea, the fourth century's version of William Osler.[10] Basil grew up in privilege and was well educated, studying Hippocratic medicine in Athens before beginning a career as a lawyer and teacher of rhetoric. In 358 C.E., he experienced a spiritual awakening, gave away his inheritance, and sought a rigorous life in ascetic desert communities. Visiting monks in Egypt, Palestine, and Syria, he marveled at their holiness, but he was disappointed to find that they did not practice works of mercy, so he left the desert and reentered public life. In the city of Caesarea, Basil soon became an assistant to the bishop, administering the bishop's charities, building food pantries and soup kitchens. He sold his own possessions to purchase food for neighbors during famines and persuaded his wealthy neighbors to do the same. Basil asked his parishioners, "What keeps you from giving now? Isn't the poor person there? Aren't your own warehouses full? Isn't the reward promised?" He continued, "The command is clear: the hungry person is dying now, the naked person is freezing now, the person in debt is beaten now—and you want to wait until tomorrow? . . . The bread in your cupboard belongs to the hungry person; the coat hanging unused in your closet belongs to the person who needs it; the shoes rotting in your closet belong to the person with no shoes; the money, which you put in the bank, belongs to the poor. You do wrong to everyone you could help, but fail to help."[11]

Basil's exhortations were powerful, but it was hard to imagine following them today. Perhaps it meant walking with Franciszek as he began again, along with his fellow ill travelers, at Interfaith House. Perhaps I could have seen him get sober for the final time. Perhaps it meant picking him up from another Emergency Department six months later. Perhaps, but I never found out. I moved away from Chicago before Franciszek finished writing his story.

I do know that, almost twenty years later, I have a great deal more sympathy for the nurses and physicians I met with Franciszek. My training has given me experiences like theirs, moments when I have become the kind of person I swore on that afternoon never to become. If I remember the story of Franciszek's being shamed, it is because it was the first time I witnessed such an event, but it is also because I prefer to remember the failings of his nurses and physicians rather than my own.

The people I have shunned and shamed are nameless in my memory, but I can remember the many times when I retreated to the call room or the nurse's station or my office to complete the documentation necessary for our exchange offering rather than sit with a patient like Franciszek in all of his or her infirmity. Sitting alone, working on the stacks of paperwork that now constitute a physician's day, I realize that Basil's homily is directed at me. I do wrong to everyone I could help but fail to help.

• • •

In 370, the bishop of Caesarea died, and Basil was named his successor. Soon after being installed, Basil realized a plan he had formed while touring monastic communities as a young man. He built a *ptochotropeion*, or house for the poor, the ill, and the dispossessed, on the outskirts of Caesarea. Basil located the ptochotropeion at the edge of his city so that it would be accessible to the needy, especially travelers and strangers. In *The Birth of the Hospital in the Byzantine Empire*, the historian Timothy Miller describes the ptochotropeion as a collection of buildings housing a large number of ill people, men and women alike. When patients entered, the clerics, deacons, and deaconesses who supervised the ptochotropeion gave them rest, regular meals, and nursing care. After these disciplines were exhausted, the supervising clergy would call in the lay physicians. Physicians administered the medicines of the day in an effort to remove ill humors and, if deemed necessary, cauterized the flesh to create blisters and burns to expel ill humors.[12]

On occasion, Basil himself provided medical care at the ptochotropeion, but as bishop he was also responsible for the social welfare of the entire city, and his work as bishop prefigured contemporary public health efforts. Risse noted that in Hellenistic society, medical care was "a personal, individualized hospitalitas," chiefly offered in the homes of physicians on the basis of an individual patient's ability to pay for medical care. According to Risse, in the face of the famine and disease that often gripped an entire community and set the ill along the roads of Byzantium in search of food and respite, Hellenistic medical care was "clearly inadequate."[13] During public health crises, Hellenistic society lacked a communitarian ideology strong enough to succor the ill. Basil stepped into the breach and developed a system of social welfare and public health that ameliorated the effects of famine.

Today, many scholars consider Basil's ptochotropeion the first hospital in Western society. He is also, after a fashion, the first healthcare reformer, because his tenure inspired the building of hospitals for the indigent ill in cities throughout the West.

• • •

After I finished my work with Stanley Hauerwas and then my psychiatry residency, I wanted to see what had become of Basil's vision. I took a job at a contemporary hospital for the indigent ill. Denver Health is a direct descendant of both Basil's ptochotropeion, as a refuge for the indigent ill, and Osler's teaching wards, as a place for the wise, as Flexner's *Report* put it, to be brought to book. I never left, because it is a place that provides physicians and other practitioners daily opportunities to serve the ill while teaching students and residents to do likewise.

Still, Denver Health suffers from what Victoria Sweet noticed at Laguna Honda. Laguna Honda's purpose, to care for the ill stranger irrespective of his or her ability to pay, was defined millennia ago. But when people receive care as patients or work in these hospitals as practitioners, Sweet wrote, they follow scripts initiated by their predecessors with little awareness of how the scripts developed. Sweet drew my attention to the way the past has become an obscured "faint shadow," but remains "active in our thoughts and desires," when we practice medicine in these settings.[14]

At Denver Health, the faint shadow of Basil's desire to create a house of healing for the indigent ill is still active in the thoughts and desires of its practitioners, even though few of them know of our debt to Basil's hospital and the way it was animated by Jewish and Christian accounts of charity. I wonder how aware of the past one must be in order to sustain practices we have inherited. How long can practices endure as faint shadows? How long can we describe the hospital as a factory before we forget that it began as a poorhouse?

I sometimes ask myself these questions from the small garden in front of the hospital, where a bench was installed that I have come to regard as an emblem of this shadowed purpose. The bench is an artful half circle, cut from stone, on which the words "DO JUSTICE. LOVE GOODNESS. WALK HUMBLY." are carved. No source is named, no text cited, no mention is made of the communities that carried those words for centuries and responded to their prophetic demands. The "Micah bench" is a clue to what hospitals once were (and could still be), but I worry that if its origins remain in the shadows, physicians will forget that they are the servants of their patients. We will be more like customer service agents instead.

Smoking anywhere on hospital grounds is banned with the vigor of a religious prohibition, but patients and visitors continue to smoke in front of the hospital's most visible entrance. Their disregard of the prohibition reminds me of how the recommendations of physicians fail. Or how they backfire: Physicians used to recommend cigarettes to patients. If you look, you can easily find old advertisements claiming that dentists smoke Viceroys, but physicians smoke Camels. Camels were, physician pitchmen avowed, less irritating for the throat.[1]

In Denver, many of our hospital smokers are lighting up joints or vaping marijuana. Although smoking marijuana publicly is illegal in Colorado, the law is inconsistently enforced, and so you can often smell its oily aroma as you enter the hospital. Our local magazines carry images of physicians recommending different strains—an indica such as Blue Widow for multiple sclerosis, a sativa such as Candy Jack for cancer—which makes the possibility of physicians recommending cigarettes suddenly seem less outré. Indeed, if you ask the marijuana smokers on the Micah bench, many will tell you that a physician recommended marijuana.

Unlike the cigarette smokers, who typically look shame-faced about smoking, the marijuana smokers are often evangelistic about their own habit. They say it is the only medicine that works. They will show you their state-issued medical marijuana registry card, popularly called a "red card" because of its red border. The phrase always makes me think of soccer matches, where referees pull a red card out of their pocket to signal that a player's foul is so egregious he or she has been exiled to the bench. In Colorado, pulling a red card out of your pocket provides access to medical marijuana, granting you an affirmative defense against prosecution. These red cards keep you in the game rather than take you out of it. When I ask someone with a red card how he or she came by it, I am usually told that the patient initiated the conversation and asked the physician for marijuana. The physician served the patient's needs, but as a customer service agent.

Because their habit is medicalized, most of the marijuana smokers will happily talk with me if I find a seat on the Micah bench. Most of them would be more likely to share a joint with a physician than to pinch it out prematurely when a doctor walked by.

One of my favorite smokers was a young man who sat vigil on the Micah bench, waiting for news of his friend in the surgical ICU. Cyrus was as thin as a wind-ravaged tree in late autumn, fingering a collection of Wallace Stevens poems in his left hand while he used his right to hold a lit marijuana cigarette and absentmindedly stroke his hair.

He did not want to be called Cyrus. He had rechristened himself Fusion Mondrian. He told me that the name was originally a literary conceit, but it was such a good name that he decided to make it real. His speech-acts had that power. The name was a month old, as long as his tenure in Colorado. He had relocated from Houston the month before "to spread a creative gospel that will make the world a more interesting place." He looked like he would be more interesting company than the regulars in the hospital's cafeteria, so I sat awhile, listening to his poetic phrases.

"How have you been making out since you came to Colorado?"

"It's been electric."

"Ah, okay. How have you been supporting yourself?"

"I am an artist and aphorist."

"Much of a market for that?"

"I live on the bird's fire-fangled feathers dangling down."

"Nice line. I like Stevens too. So you sell the feathers?"

"No. I move about. When I was in Texas, Colorado was the bronze distance, like a mid-tropic zone, or better yet, a chromatic color scale that could only be explained in music, so I shuffled the moments and moved north."

"Was medical marijuana part of the attraction?"

"Sure. The weed here is Whitmanesque, like mother of pearl, leading to sudden insights of an artistic nature, then a really diverse group of tears, and finishing with an ocean at the end of the mind."

"Not palms?"

"No, an ocean. I prefer the aesthetic climate."

We have no ocean in Colorado, but Cyrus was on to something with his comment about the aesthetic climate. Colorado is an aspirational state, an idea as much as a place. My great-great-grandfather sailed from Germany to seek his fortune in a Colorado silver mine. Today, young men like Cyrus wash up on the hospital's shores every week—erstwhile English majors, coffee-shop philosophers, and secondhand romantics who chased the wild mercury in their minds to Colorado, seeking a plant rather than a precious metal (though the potential for profit is still there: marijuana was a $700 million industry in its first full year of operation).[2]

There was Marcus, who left a Roxborough, Massachusetts, group home to attend the 420 Rally in downtown Denver. He was thrilled at smoking marijuana with thousands of other enthusiasts in a park facing the state capitol, and he liked the weather, so he decided to stay. He lived on Denver's streets in the summer and moved into the shelters in the winter. He declined the hospital's offer of a bus ticket back to the Bay State, where his sister had a spare room waiting for him. He told me, "I have a red card, and it works every time I want to travel in my mind. A bus ticket works only once."

Zeke had a girlfriend in Denver who had mailed duct-taped and bubble-wrapped packages of BHO, honey-colored hash oil filtered through lighter fluid into crystallized resins, to his Wisconsin home. He loved the BHO, and he loved her, so he moved to Colorado. When he arrived, they celebrated by sampling a fresh batch, but it was too potent for Zeke. Within eight hours of his arrival in Denver, his girlfriend brought him down from Capitol Hill to the hospital, seeking medical assistance for his paranoia. She broke up with him in the Emergency Department.

While visiting from Illinois, Salvador drank grape sativa sodas with friends. The edibles—multicolored gummy bears sprayed with aerosolized hash oil, chocolate bars filled with cannabis, cane sugar sodas infused with sativa—surprise people because they look and taste like the sugared treats favored by ten-year-olds, but they pack a medicated punch. Those sodas can have 75 mg of THC, the chief psychoactive component of cannabis, so gulping a single one can be the equivalent of smoking several joints.

Three sodas in, Salvador decided to chase a blood moon down Federal Boulevard on a friend's motorcycle. When he clipped the fender of a Mustang while racing a red light, Salvador went over his handlebars, caterwauling into the warm light of a summer night. When he landed, his body splintered into a textbook of eponymous fractures—a Le Fort III fracture of his left maxilla, an Allman II fracture of his left clavicle, and a Gustilo III fracture of his left tibia and fibula. The paramedics delivered him to Accident and Emergency, the emergency physicians staunched his wounds, the surgeons soldered his bones together, and the internists treated his pneumothorax. By the time we saw him in the Psych Department, he was eager to leave the hospital and try a different strain of cannabis. When we asked him about changing his habits, all he would commit to was staying off his cousin's bike while high. He had lost his driver's license after the accident, but he still had his red card. He was still in the game.

I am young enough to sympathize with these young men. I remember wanting to light out for parts unknown and seek a life beyond familiar frontiers, and I remember settling for moving halfway across the continent to resolve relationships that were doomed before I arrived and salting my speech with lines copped from poets. I appreciate the spirit of their endeavors.

What I struggle to appreciate are the motives of the physicians who sign for their red cards.

• • •

A couple of years ago, my colleagues and I surveyed every patient admitted to our inpatient unit for a year. We found that by their own report, our patients are seven times more likely to have a red card than the average Coloradan.[3] The implication is debatable. Many of my patients tell me that marijuana helps them. I counter that if marijuana were as helpful as they claim, they probably would not be in the hospital, that there is very little evidence for using marijuana as a medicine, but there are stacks of scientific papers showing that marijuana exacerbates mental illnesses, especially for people under the age of twenty-five.[4] But arguing is pointless. Moralizing helps no one, and I learned from writing a Cochrane review that patients often find scientific data unconvincing.

When it became clear how often we were caring for young people with red cards, we attempted to coordinate our care with that of the physicians recommending the pot. We asked patients for the names of the physicians who had recommended their marijuana, but many could not recall the physician's name, a quotidian failure in contemporary medicine. Some knew the physician's name but said that the recommending physician had asked that it be kept secret, an uncommon failure in contemporary medicine. A few patients did give us the recommending physician's name. When we called to report that a patient in the physician's practice was hospitalized and requested a call back to coordinate care, none of the physicians ever responded. Surprised, I tried to track down some of the physicians recommending medical marijuana. It proved difficult.

Like many states, Colorado keeps an online database where any physician can look up a patient and see the controlled substances—benzodiazepines, narcotics, stimulants, and the like—that a patient is receiving and who prescribed them. Although these medications are clinically useful, they are widely abused; the database helps physicians keep track of who is receiving what meds and from whom in our fractured healthcare system. In the hospital, we use the database to contact outpatient physicians to tell them that their patients are misusing or abusing the medications they prescribed. In Colorado, however, a physician recommends, rather than prescribes, medical marijuana, so the physicians who recommend marijuana are not included in the database.

I looked up the separate database kept by the state of the patients registered to use medical marijuana and the physicians who recommended marijuana to them, but the patients and physicians in this register are anonymous. While maintaining anonymity, this register discloses enough data to give a sense of big trends, including the number of red cards a physician has signed. In the past fourteen years, fifteen physicians have signed up more than half the patients, and thirty-five physicians signed up 90 percent of the patients on the state registry.[5]

The registry does not name these physicians, but you can find hints in local newspapers and magazines. Some physicians advertise their willingness to sign red cards, and some speak to the press, which has reported that these physicians have signed up people for red cards while examining them in motels, within marijuana dispensaries, or in Airstream trailers parked next to dispensaries that move daily for the convenience of patients and the discretion of the physicians. Salvador had mentioned getting his red card from a physician in an Airstream trailer flying a Red Cross flag, so I looked up the company and gave them a call. They would neither identify the physician nor allow me to leave a message seeking to coordinate care for Salvador.

• • •

Finally, I met a red card physician who would talk to me. Dr. Paul Bregman is a great talker and asked me to meet him at a restaurant near the hospital. He arrived wearing scuffed Air Jordans, baggy tweed pants, a black T-shirt, and the kind of green blazer given out to the winners of golf tournaments. He was bespectacled and paunchy but looked wonderfully alert, and as I reached out to shake his right hand he placed a bag of Ho-Hos infused with cannabis into my left.

"What's this?"

"Samples. I want you to see the amazing."

"You know, I was hoping for the lunch special."

He took the Ho-Hos back and as the hostess walked us to our table started talking. He was generous with his story. He was a radiologist who used to be in academic medicine, training residents to identify subtle lesions and flaws in the body. Long hours. Nights on call fragmenting his sleep. He became manic—the full fire—and spent years in treatment. He needed electroconvulsive therapy to compose himself, but he still could not reclaim his previous equanimity. He stopped practicing medicine and went on disability. He had climbed Osler's ladder, and then fallen off. After he had spent months purposelessly puttering, a friend introduced him to marijuana, which helped him endure being disabled and losing his social status as a physician. When medical marijuana was allowed in Colorado, he dusted off his medical license and started recommending it to other sufferers for a fee.

I asked him how the system worked. He said that patients seeking marijuana came to him. Most patients who found him had used pot before, but some were novices, curious to see whether marijuana would work better than conventional treatments. Some patients had multiple sclerosis or cancer, but most had nagging injuries and old ailments that had never been resolved with other treatments. I asked whether he performed physical examinations (something few radiologists do), and he laughed. He said that he was an expert, but not in the physical examination, and he did not see the need for an examination anyway. By listening to a patient's story (another skill in which radiologists receive scant training), he claimed that he could discern what kind of marijuana the person needed.

He told me that he assumed other physicians had examined his patients, and he encouraged patients to bring in their medical records; he saw his own role as a kind of consultant. He spoke with patients for ten or fifteen minutes and recommended a marijuana strain, a mechanism of delivery, a dose, and a frequency. He rarely saw patients for return visits, encouraging them to follow up with their regular physicians. He wished more medical marijuana physicians would do a better job of coordinating the patient's care, but he admitted that he did not initiate coordination-of-care conversations with physicians like me.

As the meal went on, I enjoyed his enthusiasm and sympathized with his situation, but I worried about his imprudence. He had described himself as an expert in a practice for which his radiology training had not prepared him: a practice where he saw patients one time, performed no examination, and then recommended a single treatment—marijuana. He told me that although he also recommended lifestyle changes, he prescribed no other medications. He admitted that he knew more about marijuana than he did about his patients' physical exam, but his patients paid in cash and left the visits happy. I asked about complications—what did he suggest for patients, such as Zeke, who became paranoid? He confidently stated that high doses of sugar could alleviate any psychosis, a claim I wished Archie Cochrane had been at the table to hear. I asked whether he thought that marijuana was simply a form of patent medicine, in which every possible ailment—the list he rattled off included dementia, diabetes, fibromyalgia, hepatitis C, psoriasis, and rheumatoid arthritis—would respond to the same prescription. He laughed and said I did not understand. He felt better on marijuana. His patients felt better on marijuana. His patients wanted marijuana. He provided what they wanted.

• • •

I spend my days navigating the gaps between what patients want and what I recommend. On any given week, I might meet a woman who has almost killed herself using a particular medicine but becomes angry when I refuse to prescribe the same medicine to her at discharge, or a man who abuses alcohol who wants me to sign him up for disability instead of rehab. I receive these kinds of requests as misdirected statements of need. The patients are certainly in need, but they are usually demoralized and are taking the simplest way out of their situation, even if that way is contrary to their health.

Society grants physicians and other medical practitioners the ability to bend the rules of the social order. We can bend the rules toward justice or toward self-interest, and we have a great deal of latitude in deciding what the difference is. In Colorado, a radiologist can, without performing a mental or physical examination, give a patient permission to grow, possess, and use dozens of marijuana plants. More prosaically, physicians like me can prescribe medications for almost any indication, write letters excusing patients from work or school or in support of a disability claim, testify that a particular act was a willful crime or an unintended action motivated by mental illness, and declare a person fit or unfit to manage his or her own finances. Physicians authorize patients' access to medications, procedures, and social roles that are otherwise unavailable.

In his classic study *The Social System*, the sociologist Talcott Parsons argued that societies grant authority to physicians and patients through what he calls the "sick role." Every culture constructs illness differently, but Parsons observed that, in its broad contours, every culture has an account of how a person enters the social role of being a patient. In the sick role, a patient is exempted from normal social responsibilities. A patient is excused from class or work or familial obligations because he or she is sick. A patient is considered sick because of something beyond the control of his or her own will. A person who is sick cannot become well simply by deciding to be or by learning a new skill. But a patient who is sick is expected to want to get well. Patients are allowed the sick role only if they are committed to doing what they can to leave it. Finally, a patient is expected to seek "technically competent help" and to cooperate with that help. A patient is expected to depend upon others, including physicians and other practitioners.[6]

Within the sick role, physicians have obligations, just as patients do. For Parsons, the chief obligation of a physician is to be an altruistic professional whose behavior is governed by the ethics of the medical profession, not by self-interest. Parsons had a particular moral version of the physician in mind, a universalized image shaped by the Protestant faith of his childhood. His description of a physician as an altruistic professional who embodies universal and neutral collective ideals was published in 1951, and it can seem outmoded today. Physicians and patients no longer share the social consensus—about what it means to be ill, to seek medical assistance, or to administer medical assistance—that Parsons was able to assume in the middle of the twentieth century.

It seems that one consequence of the loss of social consensus has been the rise of the quality-improvement movement, whose adherents distrust the professional ethics Parsons could assume operated. Because we no longer agree on what it means to be a professional, we instead pursue standardized outcomes through industrial processes perfected by quality-improvement advocates.

What seems peculiar to me is that even after we lost our shared sense of the physician's role, we not only preserved our view of the patient's social role, we extended it. Over the past fifty years, we have expanded the sick role so that conditions once considered a part of everyday existence are now considered illnesses. An aging man is urged to rub testosterone cream on his shoulders, while a woman with visible hair on her lips applies eflornithine cream twice daily, both treatments requiring a physician's prescription. The sick role remains the doorway to many changes in social circumstances, and physicians open that door.

Opening that door can, in many instances, be very lucrative for physicians.

The popular press documents stories of "pill mills," practices where physicians prescribe controlled substances such as benzodiazepines, narcotics, and stimulants for inappropriate indications at unsound amounts for obscene profits. These physicians become, like slaves in Aristotle's formulation, the animated tools of their patients' desires. Unlike Aristotle's slaves, however, they can become quite wealthy, trading their privileged access to restricted treatments for money.

Pill mills are pilloried with such vigor that I suspect we offer them up as sacrifices for the rest of medicine's sins. After all, even physicians who operate legal practices do so in an environment where the rules governing their practice have undergone startling changes since Parsons's time.

In *Remaking the American Patient: How Madison Avenue and Modern Medicine Turned Patients into Consumers*, the historian Nancy Tomes revealed how changes since Parson's era have turned patients into consumers and most physicians into customer service agents. One change Tomes identified was the lifting of the prohibition against advertising medical services. It was long considered unprofessional to advertise medical services, and before 1982, the American Medical Association formally forbade physicians to advertise. Fifteen years later, the Food and Drug Administration allowed pharmaceutical companies to begin advertising directly to the public. Today, physicians, hospitals, insurers, and pharmaceutical companies advertise their wares in every possible setting. Tomes identified their ability to do so, based on the rise of market research and the advertising industry, as an additional change. Market researchers and advertisers turned healthy but anxious people into patients and patients into consumers; they created a need for a medical product or intervention, and then filled the need with a new pill or cream or procedure. Advertisers championed the "rights" of consumers to receive their brand-name treatments at brand-name prices. Now we live in a world where physicians, hospitals, insurers, and pharmaceutical companies all conceal their failures from public view but trumpet their successes with the techniques of contemporary advertising.[7]

Those techniques have altered our daily lives in many ways. Consider just one metric, the use of prescription drugs: two-thirds of Americans now take a medication available to them only with a physician's prescription. Americans spend twice as much on pharmaceutical medications as they spend on new automobiles. And one outcome of this is that twice as many American are killed by prescription medications as are killed in automobile accidents every year.[8]

The effects on the practice of medicine are perverse. Pharmaceutical companies direct the majority of their advertising efforts to the people who can open the door to their profitable treatments; for every six American physicians, there is one pharmaceutical salesperson. Physicians who are frequent prescribers are groomed and detailed by pharmaceutical corporations to increase prescriptions of profitable pharmaceuticals. In my own specialty of psychiatry, some psychiatrists describe themselves as "psychopharmacologists," as if they ministered to medications rather than to patients.

I know a psychiatrist who describes himself this way. He also routinely shows up on the lists of physicians who receive tens of thousands of dollars a year from pharmaceutical companies in exchange for promoting their medications. A few years ago, I admitted a string of his patients to the unit, all of whom had decompensated after he switched them to a new medication whose manufacturer was paying for him to give talks around town. I called him and shared my concern; he offered to bring lunch to the hospital and meet with me. I agreed, assuming that two physicians could work out their differences over a collegial meal.

When I entered the conference room where we were to meet, I realized that he had come with a lunch paid for by the manufacturer of the new medication. As I walked in the door, he offered me a box lunch and a handshake, then began clicking his way through a slide deck prepared by the manufacturer of, coincidentally, the same medication for which I had previously written a Cochrane review. A few years previously I had sifted through all the published and unpublished data on the same drug. While writing the Cochrane review required two years of unpaid labor, this physician was being paid to deliver me an hour-long speech about its benefits written by the manufacturer. I had to admit that his presentation was more exciting than our review, if decidedly less systematic.

I left the unopened box lunch on the conference room table a few minutes later. As near as I could tell, he was as self-interested as the pot-permitting radiologist, but not as cheerful.

Back on the ward, I ran into a fellow physician who had skipped the lunch, having scoped out the intent more quickly than I. He thought me naive and the drug-repping physician cheap. He joked that if you are going to use your medical license for the benefit of a large corporation, you should become your own for-profit corporation. He proposed an openly criminal exchange, an offshore website that would provide electronically signed prescriptions for Xanax, Fentanyl, or Ambien to anyone willing to pay with a valid credit card. He did some quick calculations and figured out that if he could keep it up for six months, he could retire young from medicine. Until such a tax shelter is in place, though, he decided to continue practicing workaday medicine, seeing one patient at a time.

• • •

We call them by that contested term *patients*. Each patient is a person, irreducibly complex and particular, but when I meet hospitalized people, I welcome them as patients, as people in Parsons's sick role. They have responsibilities as patients, and I have responsibilities to them as a physician. These responsibilities are often obscured, but they remain accessible.

Years ago, Stanley Hauerwas taught me that for all of medicine's problems, we can still find reminders of its shadowed purpose in its language. So when we call physicians, and other practitioners, professionals, Hauerwas says we are drawing upon a memory of the original idea of the profession as "a calling for a special service to the common good." Similarly, he claimed that one moral significance of calling ill people "patients" is that it reminds us of the virtue of patience, of persevering through the inevitable diminishments, sufferings, and losses of human existence. He advised all future patients—all of us, really—to practice patience before we inevitably become sick.[9]

But this sounds difficult. If one could choose, who would choose patient suffering over immediate relief? Who is willing to wait when he or she is simply inconvenienced, let alone when his or her health is imperiled?

The contemporary Dutch philosopher Annemarie Mol recently wrote that ill people are best understood as patients precisely because no one would choose illness, frailty, diminishment, and death. Like Hauerwas, Mol observed that although we talk in contemporary medicine about making health choices and choosing treatment options, this language misses the reality of our lives. Our lives are concerned with making do with the bodies we have rather than choosing better bodies. Mol made this observation in her quietly profound *The Logic of Care: Health and the Problem of Patient Choice*, which developed out of careful observation of patients and medical practitioners in a diabetes clinic in the Netherlands. In the clinic she found, within the languages and practices of patients and practitioners, two competing logics.

The first logic, the logic of choice, was adopted as a corrective to the paternalism of medicine. We gave up one cliché, the doctor knows best, in favor of another, the customer is always right. Mol observed that when we imagine ill people using this logic, we alternately imagine them as consumers choosing medical services on a healthcare market or citizens entering into contracts with healthcare providers. Although these models have distinct registers, Mol observed that both emphasize an ill person's ability to make a choice for his or her health. Emphasizing choice appeals to our contemporary interest in using market-based reforms to achieve efficiency and effectiveness, but Mol observed that fostering patient choice has eroded preexisting practices established to ensure good care. Choice cannot account for the realities of living with a diseased body. We cannot purchase health as we can other products, nor can we enter into a contract that will guarantee predictable outcomes from our unpredictable bodies. The only predictable outcome of life is that we will die, a reality from which the logic of choice intentionally distracts customers. In the logic of choice, professionals enable this distraction by limiting their role to the presentation of facts and the use of instruments to enact the choices made by an ill person.

The second logic, the logic of care, harks back to an older language, in which ill people were understood as patients. In this logic, an ill person is not constituted either by his or her choices or by an ability or inability to make those choices but by the practices in which he or she engages while adapting to living with illness. In this conception, making treatment decisions is one among many practices, not the practice that gives a person his or her identity. The question is how to live with and within our bodies. The logic of choice promises mastery over the body, so what matters to an ill person is who masters the body and what outcomes are achieved. The logic of care is less concerned with outcomes because what matters is whether or not someone cares for you. From professionals, the logic of care requires patience, mutual respect, and the ability to take nothing for granted. Patients must admit their own frailty, vulnerability, and suffering. Patients are actively involved in tenaciously adapting to a life with illness, which demands energy and determination.[10]

If Tomes showed me how advertisers and markets taught patients to understand themselves as consumers and physicians to understand themselves as customer service agents, Mol showed me how these changes altered medical practice. When we understood ill people as customers, we altered the social relationship of illness. We neglected the ways that our lives are contingent, dependent upon circumstances beyond our control. When we became focused on choosing our own medical treatments, we forgot that we live in bodies that grow, love, weaken, and die. Mol is bracingly clear-eyed about our mortality and that our bodies are pleasurable but fragile.

The moral act in the logic of choice is making a choice. The moral act in the logic of care is practical activities. Choice is a discrete activity with a beginning and an end. Care is an open-ended process. Choice is a transaction. Care is a relationship. Choice promises outcomes. Care promises only presence. Choice tames or transcends the body. Care occurs only with the body. Choice asks who is in charge of the body. Care asks how we live with the body. Choice assumes that scientific knowledge is becoming ever more certain. Care attunes scientific knowledge to particular patients. Choice is about managing the body. Care is about doctoring the body.

Mol used *doctoring* in a particular way, to describe the adaptations we make to our particular situations, with all their contingencies. She did not limit doctoring to the work of physicians, or even of other medical practitioners, but extended it to everyone who cares for the body. She wanted all of us, patient, professional, and otherwise, to engage in the experience and experiment of doctoring, of practically tinkering with the body. Mol asked us to renew the language of professional and patient, which is threatened by the marketing-sanctioned language of choice, to remind us of our shared frailties and vulnerabilities.

• • •

A few years ago, a government regulator decided that our unit would be more customer-friendly if the treatment plans, which we create with each patient when he or she is admitted to the hospital, included the stated goals of the patients. The regulator's forms forced me to record whatever goals a patient identified. For a week, I wrote down goals like "to finish the suicide I started," "to get the moon to stop bothering me," and "to change the United States Constitution so that the FBI has direct authority over the CIA." Each patient insisted that these phrases best described his or her treatment goals.

Writing out these goals helped, in a fashion. I was able to convince the regulator that repeating patients' goals verbatim would not work on the unit. It also made it clear to me that I am not in the business of customer service. I will not complete a patient's botched suicide. I have no power over the moon, to say nothing of the Constitution. I could not help patients meet these goals.

And yet I could sit with each patient and listen to him or to her, so that we could try, together, to find a common rhythm where we could find the logic of care. Even the regulators have evidence for the benefit of a common rhythm. In a report, the Joint Commission, the leading regulator of medicine, attributed more than two-thirds of all serious adverse events in hospitals to failures of communication.[11] So perhaps we could all agree that physicians and patients should try to rediscover those common rhythms. With Cyrus, finding a common rhythm meant talking in words borrowed from a Wallace Stevens poem. I would not be his customer service agent, but, perhaps I could be a witness to his experience as we sat together on the Micah bench.

It always surprises me what people will reveal to a physician. Every day, I introduce myself to strangers, and they answer my personal questions, even the most probing. I ask where they live and with whom, whom they love, with whom they lie down, how they make and spend money, and what they hope for in the future. When physicians ask the right questions, people answer.

Jonah answered our questions, but only after being attended to through the logic of care. Not that Jonah spoke. Jonah answered our questions, but I never heard him say a word.

I met Jonah during my residency. He was eleven years old. When I met him, he had already been refraining from speech for three months, and he would remain silent for three more. While Jonah was silent, I spoke to anyone who would speak to me, and I gathered every record I could find of when Jonah had spoken to physicians.

When we unfolded Jonah's medical records on a table in the nurse's lounge, each text was fragmented, beginning mid-thought and ending without resolution, with more aporias and erasures than a postmodern novel. The authors of these texts—ever changing, for the same physician rarely saw Jonah twice—always deferred diagnosis until after a new test or study was procured from another physician. No physician saw a result from all these efforts; diagnosis was the ever distant horizon.

Looking at the gathered charts, we reconstructed a history. Jonah was conceived in poverty, the last child of a family fissured by illness and substance abuse. When not drunk, his father, Matta, was encouraging. When not depressed, his mother, Deb, was caring. Deb had many reasons for her frequent dysphoria. She supported herself through public assistance and sex work. She did not know the fathers of several of her children. Some of her children lived with her, some with her parents, and some were in foster care.

After birth, Jonah was hospitalized in a neonatal intensive care unit with pulmonary edema. He went "home" two weeks later. Sometimes he lived with his mother and sometimes with her parents. We sketched out his family tree—it was twisted in on itself because two of Jonah's half-siblings had a child together—and included the known diagnoses of each family member. The number of diagnoses increased as we worked down the generations, and the diseases listed read like the table of contents of a health inequality textbook; they included bipolar disorder, diabetes, fibromyalgia, hepatitis C, major depressive disorder, pancreatitis, and schizophrenia.[1] By the time the family tree reached Jonah's generation, the names of adolescents were often wreathed by five or more chronic illnesses.

Except for Jonah's name. He had remained healthy enough to avoid physicians. He enjoyed reading and was a good student, earning As and Bs. He kept his grades up even when, at the age of seven, he entered foster care after his maternal grandfather, Floyd, was convicted of sexual assault on a woman. In foster care, Jonah received counseling but no psychotropic medications or diagnoses, a surprising circumstance because foster children are often overmedicated and overdiagnosed with psychiatric illnesses.[2] Two years later, Matta sobered up, won custody of Jonah, and took him out of foster care. They shared a modest house, but it was their own.

When Floyd was released from prison a year later, he moved in across the street and helped out. Over the next year, Jonah began seeking the help available to him. He entered the sick role. Around his tenth birthday, he began showing up at the Emergency Department near his home. He came in with vague complaints. A subjective fever. Occasional diarrhea. Back pain. Choking episodes. Throat pain. He told one physician, "I strain my brain to think." An MRI was ordered. A bone scan. Both examinations were "unremarkable," which is the euphemism we physicians use when we suspect something is broken but cannot quite see where. Jonah was sent home with a large bill for services rendered, but without a diagnosis.

Over the following summer, Jonah gradually stopped walking. First he borrowed a cane from his grandfather Floyd. Then two canes. Then a wheelchair. His parents were concerned enough to return to the Emergency Department, despite the cost. After one visit, for wheezing and painful swallowing, Jonah was hospitalized overnight and received a fistful of medications—albuterol, dexamethasone, diphenhydramine, and epinephrine—that only marginally improved the wheezing. The physicians sent him home the next day with a provisional diagnosis of "spasmodic croup vs. somatization vs. malingering"; no diagnosis at all.

At home again, Jonah stopped attending school. Someone filed a report on the family with Social Services, alleging assaults by the adults on the children and by the older children on the younger children. Twice, the Department of Social Services checked in on Jonah's family. Twice, the caseworkers could not substantiate the reports, so Jonah stayed at home. His silence began soon after these visits.

His parents took him to a local pediatrician, who ordered procedures to look at his throat, a direct laryngoscopy and rigid bronchoscopy; these examinations were equally "unremarkable."

Jonah was sent home again. So that someone could be with him at night, Jonah began to share a bed with Floyd. In Jonah's family, this was part of the sick role. Whenever Jonah had been sick as a small child, he had slept in Floyd's bed. Floyd began offering Jonah liquid nutritional supplements, which he had brought home from one of his own hospitalizations. Despite their sweet flavor and gentle texture, Jonah declined the Ensures. He ate and drank less each day.

Four weeks later, Jonah's parents carried him again to the Emergency Department. The emergency physician rehydrated him with intravenous fluids and diagnosed Jonah with failure to thrive, hysterical stridor, and perioral abrasions. The physician suspected a psychiatric problem, so he referred Jonah to a community mental health center.

Jonah and Matta went once to the community mental health center. They left with a prescription for fluoxetine, a drug to increase his available serotonin, but they never filled it and never returned.

A week later, Jonah was hospitalized for pain with swallowing so severe he was refusing all food. Once admitted, the medical staff reported that he only sipped juice and ate ice chips. Consulting psychiatrists prescribed mirtazapine to increase his appetite and improve his mood, but Jonah refused the medication. Pediatricians observed that he spit up half of every meal and diagnosed him with anorexia nervosa, a diagnosis that described Jonah's behavior without explaining it.

Physicians ordered more tests. A pharyngeal function study. An otolaryngologist consult. The physicians were still looking for a broken part while Jonah was silently fading away. The physicians threaded a nasogastric tube into Jonah's stomach, taped it in place, and began feeding Jonah pureed meals.

Finally, a new pediatrician joined the team, and she looked again at Jonah. She tested a sample of Jonah's urine and found chlamydia. She treated Jonah with antibiotics for chlamydia and, since they often travel together, a presumed gonorrhea infection. She asked Jonah if she could swab his urethra to see exactly which bacteria were present, but Jonah refused. With the pediatrician's encouragement, though, he opened his silent mouth long enough for her to swab his pharynx. The sample grew gonorrhea. The inquisitive pediatrician recalled that Jonah had been sharing a bed with his grandfather and asked to speak alone with Jonah's grandmother, who admitted that Floyd had a history of sexually transmitted infections.

The pediatrician called the police. A few days later, she transferred Jonah to our psychiatric hospital. When he was wheeled in, he was eleven years old, weighed sixty-six pounds, and did not eat, talk, or walk independently.

• • •

When we talk about reforming medicine by restructuring it around the needs of customers, I think of patients like Jonah.

On one hand, his experience points to many of the failures of our systems. He was seen by multiple physicians, who did not consult with one another, were trained to examine only specific parts of his body, ordered numerous expensive tests and procedures, recorded their findings in incomprehensible medical records, and never integrated the results into a comprehensive account of Jonah's condition. These physicians engaged in unceasing activity, most of it unnecessary and uneconomical, while Floyd continued to molest Jonah. The physicians maintained the clinical volumes and operating margins that keep our hospitals and clinics afloat but missed many opportunities to halt Jonah's decline into silent dependency.

On the other hand, I doubt that the most recent prescriptions for healthcare reform would have helped Jonah either. In these accounts, Jonah would be understood as a customer for whom healthcare providers should deliver the best outcomes. They would optimize the benefits physicians and other healthcare practitioners provided him with. In practice, that means following standardized clinical guidelines, comparable to the computerized instructions displayed at the line chefs' stations at the Cheesecake Factory, which rarely account for situations like Jonah's, and measuring outcomes by performance on quality measures that assess compliance to those guidelines rather than true outcomes of a patient's well-being. In a psychiatric hospital, the "quality" of Jonah's hospitalization would be measured by seven items, such as whether a complete list of his medications and his treatment plan were transmitted to an outpatient practitioner at discharge. These seven items are necessary but insufficient measures of whether or not we have provided the "quality" care that patients like Jonah need.[3] A psychiatric hospital could achieve perfect quality scores for Jonah's care even if it discharged him home to Floyd, because one can often meet the quality metrics without addressing the real problem.

Even if we could develop the right evidence-based guidelines and patient-centered outcome measures to enable physicians to practice medicine with impeccable customer service, another obstacle would remain: too few practitioners are willing to care for the poor, even though a sadly extensive body of literature shows that race and poverty are powerful predictors of illness.[4] Illness increases as inequality increases to the extent that, if you tell an epidemiologist your zip code, he or she can estimate how long you are likely to live.

There is another equally extensive body of literature showing that physicians and hospitals often preselect the patients who will have the best outcomes and the best reimbursements. High-skill physicians frequently seek low-risk patients to maximize their scores on quality report cards.[5] Basil built his hospital where the indigent ill lived; today's clinics and hospitals are clustered where the wealthy live. We physicians often serve the wealthy instead of the poor.

The great critic of this trend is the physician Paul Farmer, who excoriates contemporary medicine for its unjust distribution of medical services. Farmer argues that the problem is not that we do not know how to deliver the advances of contemporary medicine but that we choose the wrong people to whom we deliver the advances. It is not simply that we do not bring the meal to the table on time and at the right price; many people are never invited to the table at all. Farmer observes that by any measure the poor suffer a disproportionate share of the burdens of illness, and he insists that they ought therefore to receive a disproportionate share of the benefits of medicine. Medicine could be renewed, Farmer wrote in *Pathologies of Power: Health, Human Rights, and the New War on the Poor*, if physicians and other practitioners engaged in "pragmatic solidarity . . . delivered with dignity to the destitute sick" instead of customer service.[6]

For Farmer, a medical practice seeking "pragmatic solidarity" would consist of observing, judging, and acting. By observing, Farmer meant identifying the social and economic conditions that limit the agency of the poor and imperil their health. By judging, Farmer meant identifying the structures that inflict suffering upon the poor. Finally, by acting, Farmer meant the obligation of medicine to redress the suffering of the poor. Farmer wants justice rather than charity for the indigent ill.[7]

In contrast, noted Farmer, conventional medicine usually consists of preventing, treating, and curing. Farmer admired these activities but lamented that they were unable to identify and act against the underlying economic and political causes of suffering. So he disparaged medicine as consumerist while envisioning its renewal, writing, "In a world riven by inequity, medicine could be viewed as a social justice work. In fact, doctors are far more fortunate than most modern professionals: we still have a sliver of hope for meaningful, dignified service to the oppressed. Few other disciplines can make this claim with any honesty."[8]

And few other physicians are capable of making this claim with more rhetorical currency than Paul Farmer, because few physicians have so fully realized their commitments. When Farmer wrote that "pragmatic solidarity" demands making the best contemporary medicine available to the destitute ill before making these resources available to the privileged ill, he was describing his own work. With colleagues, Farmer founded Partners in Health, a nongovernmental organization that extends the advances of contemporary medicine to the poor in countries as diverse as Haiti, Malawi, Peru, and Russia. Where other agencies have declared that it is impractical to deliver the best care in such impoverished locales, Partners in Health has repeatedly proven them wrong by pioneering methods that bring excellent care to the poor.

They do so not by imposing a model developed by corporate headquarters that is exported to the local franchises of biomedicine but by building partnerships with local organizations. They resemble CrossFit more than the Cheesecake Factory. The name of Partners in Health is literal—Farmer and his colleagues believe we must be "partners" with local communities and with the poor. The organization's mission is, simply, "to provide a preferential option for the poor in health care."[9]

Farmer developed the idea of being a partner to the poor, and of seeking a preferential option for the poor, from his encounters with the Peruvian priest Gustavo Gutiérrez. Gutiérrez is a Dominican, like those with whom I volunteered in Chicago, and a pioneering liberation theologian. Developed in Latin American communities in the 1950s and 1960s, liberation theology asserts that God is especially engaged with the poor, and church and social structures must thus be reoriented to serve the poor first. Farmer was introduced to liberation theology as an undergraduate while volunteering with a nun serving migrant farm workers. As he has said since, Farmer was drawn to liberation theology because it "does not call for equally good treatment of the poor; it demands preferential treatment for the poor." The experience led him to Haiti. He was overwhelmed by the poverty and suffering he witnessed there, but he found that liberation theology helped him "make sense of the poverty I saw around me."[10] When he subsequently attended medical school, Farmer spent most of his academic year in Haiti, living with and working alongside the indigent, helping build a clinic, and delivering medical care, then flying back to take examinations.

In Haiti, living in solidarity with the poor meant that Farmer needed to resume his practice of the Catholic faith in which he had been raised. He was not a visitor, but a partner. He found that his Catholic neighbors in Haiti were seeking justice and mercy, while many of his secular colleagues in medicine and anthropology were seeking prestige and power. Living alongside the indigent ill in Haiti as a partner, Farmer felt God's presence.

Ever since, Farmer has described liberation theology as the leavening of his medical practice and anthropological research. Liberation theology taught Farmer that to be better, to improve, required attacking poverty and inequity, the fetid conditions in which illness thrives. You must listen to the poor, not preach to them about salvation or health. You must not only treat poor patients, you must also accompany them in their struggle. He told a graduating class at Harvard's Kennedy School of Government, "To accompany someone is to go somewhere with him or her, to break bread together, to be present on a journey with a beginning and an end. . . . Accompaniment is about sticking with a task until it's deemed completed—not by the accompagnateur, but by the person being accompanied." (*Accompagnateur* is the name given by Partners in Health for community health workers who accompany their ill neighbors as they seek and receive medical care.) When you understand yourself as a partner to the poor, Farmer told the graduates, your life's work is "to accompany the destitute sick on a journey away from premature suffering and death."[11]

• • •

To accompany the destitute sick is a mighty task that most of us, even on our best days, have trouble accomplishing. I was fortunate to see it at work in Jonah's case.

When we read Jonah's gathered medical records, it was clear that while most of his physicians had worked in the usual register—prevention, treatment, cure—they were silent about his suffering. Searching for a broken part, a bone or an organ, they said little about the culture of poverty and abuse in which he lived, the domestic version of the systemic injustice that Farmer so potently associated with illness. Prevention, treatment, and cure had not worked, so we resolved to try Farmer's prescription and observe, judge, and act on Jonah's behalf.

When the silent Jonah was wheeled into our psychiatric facility, he had already been diagnosed with a psychiatric disorder, anorexia nervosa, but we always reconsider the initial psychiatric diagnosis. Although he had surely altered his eating habits and subsequently lost a significant amount of weight, his weight loss was precipitous rather than insidious, and he was preoccupied with throat pain rather than body image. Jonah's behavior had begun not because he disliked his body, but because his grandfather had invaded it. When a person who suffers trauma develops a mental illness, it is most commonly depression or posttraumatic stress disorder. Although Jonah's affect was often constricted and he exhibited ambivalence toward his own well-being, he exhibited depressive symptoms only on a situational basis. And though he occasionally had difficulty initiating sleep, he shook his head when we asked if he was having the intrusive thoughts and nightmares characteristic of posttraumatic stress disorder.

Jonah had not suffered the classic version of trauma, a discrete moment in which his life was imperiled by a violent attack or an abrupt explosion during which he believed he would die. He had suffered what some psychiatrists call complex trauma. For children, complex trauma is the experience of multiple traumatic events in interpersonal relationships throughout their developmental history.[12] Jonah's caregivers repeatedly exposed him to a variety of traumas, including hunger, shifting parental figures, poverty, physical abuse, and sexual abuse.

A child who suffers complex trauma can develop dysfunction in every aspect of his life, and while we considered other possibilities, we ultimately saw Jonah's symptoms as a kind of somatization, the bodily experience of an emotional state.[13] We all somaticize at one time or another, experiencing a discouraging remark as a headache, a difficult conversation as a stomachache, or a disappointing reversal as a backache. Since Jonah's somatization was profound enough to threaten his life, we diagnosed him with a conversion disorder, an alteration of his motor function that was incompatible with a recognized medical or neurological disorder. If he could resolve his emotional state, his legs could walk, his stomach could digest food, and his vocal cords could produce speech. But since he could not do so, he converted the unresolvable into a series of physical deficits. The term "conversion" entered the language of physicians through Freud's classic studies of hysteria, but it is the elegant formulation of the British psychiatrist Henry Maudsley—"The sorrow which has no vent in tears may make other organs weep"—that expresses why someone like Jonah somaticizes.[14]

In psychoanalytic theory, somatization is accounted as an immature defense mechanism, and children often somaticize. So pediatricians and parents are accustomed to asking about physical complaints as a way to assess the emotional state of a child.

Confusion often arises, though, because many episodes of somatization follow a physical problem; the well-intentioned care they received when ill encourages children to somaticize. For Jonah, the concerned attention of medical practitioners and his parents encouraged somatization all the way to dependency. As he declined into somatization, Jonah acquired medical supplies. After he stopped walking, he rode in a wheelchair. After he stopped eating, pediatricians snaked a nasogastric tube into his stomach. But as he stopped speaking, he needed something that could not be found in a hospital supply closet. He needed someone to speak on his behalf.

Because we believed that Jonah's sorrow was related to his trauma, we began our care of Jonah by judging who could (and who could not) see him. Floyd was free on bond, but we forbade contact. We met with each member of his family to determine who would be willing to accompany Jonah as he pursued health and justice.

Matta proved to be Jonah's best partner, but he needed assistance of his own. He had been absent during Jonah's early childhood, and even though he had lived with Jonah for the previous two years, Matta admitted that he was often distant. The psychologist taught him to relate to Jonah. The social worker found him a place to stay near the hospital, and Matta began visiting daily to speak with Jonah and the team. Even though he was still not speaking, Jonah brightened in Matta's presence. The hospital became the place where Jonah and his father became reacquainted.

As their relationship grew stronger, our treatment team met daily to discuss Jonah and make certain we provided consistent treatment. The team included the full complement of professionals available in a contemporary academic medical center—attorneys, nurses, nutritionists, occupational therapists, pediatricians, physical therapists, psychiatrists, psychologists, speech therapists, and teachers. Jonah initially responded to this treatment team with oppositional behavior and refused our interventions. He disliked the physicians, like me, who encouraged him to eat, speak, and walk. He disliked the nurses who enforced the unit's rules and measured the vital signs that signaled his physical well-being. He disliked the social workers who encouraged him to consider another foster care placement.

But he loved a psychology student who read to him. She would visit the unit in the charged quiet that followed the physicians' rounds. While the nurses and physicians were occupied with updating the electronic medical record, the student would visit Jonah in his room, pull a chair up to his hospital bed and read Harry Potter books out loud. Page after page, chapter after chapter, she read to Jonah about an orphaned child raised by a neglectful relatives who learned, on his eleventh birthday, that he was actually a wizard. Jonah's grandfather had forbidden Harry Potter books as devilish, but Jonah thawed in the warm concern of the story and the constant company of the psychology student.

Toward the end of the first month of his hospitalization, he began to accumulate advances, though they came fitfully. Following each advance, there would be a regression. The staff would reassure him, and within a few days he would progress again. He progressed from a wheelchair to a walker to a cane to holding hands with staff to walking on his own. He ate his first solid meal in five months from the hands of an occupational therapist, and two weeks later he was alternating nasogastric feeds with a regular pediatric diet; when he spontaneously vomited his nasogastric tube during an occupational therapy session, the tube was never replaced.

Meanwhile, Jonah received therapy from a trauma nurse. She would visit him independent of the team. She spent two weeks simply building a therapeutic alliance. Then she worked to help him relate his emotions to his physical experiences. When he made somatic complaints by grabbing at his stomach or pointing at his throat, she used fantasy action figures and metaphors like "growing pains" to discuss his emotional state. She instituted a token economy that allowed Jonah to begin controlling his immediate environment. He started writing to her with pencil and paper, asking about his safety.

I witnessed much of this, but I never heard Jonah speak because I rotated off the service before he started talking. Friends of mine who heard him told me that his speech returned two and a half months into the hospitalization. He started with cries, inarticulate grunts, and monosyllabic responses. His written questions to the staff became pointed, asking where he would be sent once he started speaking. Jonah met with the attorney who was prosecuting his grandfather. Jonah met with the social worker, who promised discharge to a therapeutic foster home. Jonah met with the trauma nurse, who agreed to provide intensive outpatient psychiatric follow-up at the foster home and, eventually, Matta's home. Jonah met with Matta, who promised daily visits, his own sobriety, and Jonah's safety.

Now Jonah spoke freely. He asked for books, pizza, and time off the unit with Matta.

Jonah spoke only after his team left behind prevention, treatment, and cure in favor of witnessing his suffering and committing to protect him from further suffering. After he was assured of justice, Jonah said his good-byes out loud and walked off the unit on his own.

• • •

In medicine, we are often intimate witnesses to profound suffering. We see every day how poverty, neglect, and abuse distort the bodies and minds of the people we meet as patients. We see how the poor receive profoundly different care from the rich, how they age early and die young.

We grow accustomed to such sights.

On psych units, insurers and regulators advise discharge from the hospital when patients are "stable," a euphemism meaning that a patient can survive outside the hospital. I often discharge patients to situations where bare survival is all I can offer and any hopes for an end to suffering can only be called modest. I rarely accompany people to justice and mercy.

So I am grateful that I saw, with Jonah, what medicine can achieve. I am grateful to all the practitioners, with their various skills, who were witnesses to Jonah for months, long after the reimbursements for his care stopped. These practitioners, mostly women, patiently cared for Jonah, and in doing so they showed what real improvement in healthcare looks like when practitioners heed Farmer's call to observe, judge, and act on behalf of a patient. Too often, we forget what medicine can do, but as Farmer also observed, our most costly failures are often failures of imagination.

When I feel especially discouraged by medicine, I make a list of what a reimagined medicine would look like, a medicine where physicians and other practitioners could get to know people intimately, bear witness to the social injustices they suffer, and accompany them to health and justice. On a locked psychiatric unit, my list includes the end of coercive treatment, a shared table where staff and patients could eat together, meetings between inpatient and outpatient teams, and ways to reintegrate patients into the lives of families and local communities. When I am fool enough to share my list with a regulator or administrator, he or she will look at me as if I am as daft as the patients. They know that nothing on my list is paid for by insurers or required by regulators, so they think it impossible. But I know that everything on my list is possible.

Quality-improvement advocates like to talk about battleships staffed by young workers with modest experience and skill who achieve reliable outcomes. I prefer to talk about the Mennonite Mental Health Movement, a group of young workers with comparably modest experience and skill, but more expansive imaginations.

The Mennonites are a small Anabaptist community committed to nonresistance, or meeting violence with nonviolence. Mennonites will not serve on a battleship, but they will perform alternate service in wartime.

During World War II, some fifteen hundred Mennonites performed alternative service in state psychiatric hospitals as members of the Civilian Public Service. Instead of serving in combat, they served in hospitals that were, like the Dorothea Dix Hospital at which I trained, sprawling, crowded facilities. During the war, so many on the staff of these facilities were drafted that in some instances a single staff member was left responsible for a thousand patients. The remaining staff, before the advent of effective psychotropic medicines, and without the imagination for pragmatic solidarity, often engaged in frank violence. They patrolled hospital halls with blackjacks, striking down agitated patients or stripping them naked and spraying them with water.

With little training or experience, Mennonite volunteers joined these wards and found ways to care for agitated patients without violence. On these understaffed units, Mennonites pioneered noncoercive techniques for the care of persons with mental illness.

After the war ended, Mennonite veterans were released from the Civilian Public Service, but many of them decided to build an alternative system of mental health facilities across the United States. These eight facilities directly served people with mental illness. Mennonites worked with leading psychiatrists from the National Institutes of Mental Health to provide state-of-the-art care, just as Farmer does through Partners in Health, as well as the caring environment of a Mennonite family. Forming therapeutic relationships was a part of the treatment, so at most of the facilities staff shared a common table with patients. Near at least one of the facilities, local Mennonites opened their homes to families visiting patients. The facilities also educated members of the Mennonite community about what it means to live with a mental illness and served as places for direct encounters between the indigent ill and the wealthy well. Mennonites provided the evidence-based treatments of contemporary medicine, not in pursuit of consistent outcomes but out of a pragmatic solidarity with the ill and a reimagined sense of medicine.

When the Mennonites reimagined mental healthcare through the lenses of discipleship and nonresistance, or when Paul Farmer called for medicine to become pragmatic solidarity, they were following the example of Basil.

Farmer called his peers to leave consumer medicine, where those who can pay the most receive the best care, and practice a liberating hospitality in which the poor will receive the best care and receive it first. The Mennonites called on psychiatric facilities to cease their coercive practices, where agitated and psychotic patients were violently oppressed, to practice a noncoercive care for persons with mental illness. Basil called physicians to abandon their Hellenistic medicine, where care was provided only to relatives and associates who could afford the physician's fee, and tend to the poor stranger.

All became witnesses who observed, judged, and acted in the face of injustice. They both provided exemplary medical treatment and saw that not every problem a person brings to a physician is best understood as a medical problem. Some problems will not be solved by

biomedical solutions. The Mennonites accomplished something—
providing inpatient mental health services to persons with mental
illness without using coercive measures—that still seems impossible
in most psychiatric facilities, even though we now have dozens of
effective medications. The Mennonites had none of these medicines
when they began their own efforts, but what they had was enough
imagination to look beyond evidence-based outcomes. They had alternative, communal practices of reimagined care. They bore witness in an active sense. They told stories to actuate change in the
lives of people like Jonah, so that people like Jonah could write their
own stories.

sixteen

HOPE

Eleanor was my favorite patient in residency, even though she fired me over and over again. Each time, as she returned only to fire me again, I wondered if I was the wrong physician for her or whether we were simply hoping for different results.

I first met Eleanor right after completing my internship at Dix, and I was tired. Every fourth night at Dix, I had performed emergency evaluations on twenty or so patients. They lived lives of irreducible complexity, but my responsibilities were to admit, pacify, or medicate. As my internship wore on, the particular derangements of an individual became problem sets to be solved as quickly as possible so I could retreat to the call room. It reminded me of junior high algebra when the teacher would pass out work sheets with rows of equations, each with an unknown x that needed to be identified. The problems were simple, but also revelatory—the word *algebra* derives from an Arabic word that literally means a reunion—because we restored an alienated x to itself. This is where my analogy broke down, though, because as an intern, I saw many alienated people, but I was not restoring many of them to themselves.

When I met Eleanor, I wanted to solve for x and be on my way. Her family physician suspected dementia and had referred her for a cognitive function evaluation. I grabbed a preprinted dementia checklist from my office, strode to the waiting room with unearned confidence, and called out for Eleanor. Her daughter-in-law stood up, shook my hand, and gestured to a short and bespectacled eighty-year-old woman flipping indifferently through a months-old magazine.

In the exam room, she told me her story. She had lived in the United States since the 1960s, when her husband was relocated by his job, but she still thought of herself as British. Her husband had cheated on her and she had divorced him, but stayed in the States because her children considered it home. She had returned to school and become a hospice nurse, which felt as though she were closing an open set: she had been an army nurse during the Blitz. Now retired, she lived in a small house near her son. She offered these details quickly and without emotion.

I hoped the diagnosis would be just as quick and emotionless, so I started in on my questions. She had no complaints, but she allowed that she no longer enjoyed traveling because she could not recall well-known destinations and felt undone in new environments. I administered several cognitive tests—drawing clock faces, connecting series of letters and numbers in order, memorizing three objects, and the like—most of which she was unable to complete. In a way, I was relieved that all her tests pointed to dementia because naming her broken part would therefore be straightforward. The impression was reinforced when she became lost after using the clinic's bathroom. When I brought her back to the exam room, I asked Eleanor to undergo laboratory tests to exclude correctable causes of cognitive problems. I handed her another preprinted checklist for laboratory tests. Across the top was her name, her date of birth, and the reason I was ordering the tests: "rule out organic causes of dementia."

When Eleanor saw *dementia* on the laboratory form she shouted, "How dare you use that word to describe me. Using that word to describe me is like calling a black person a nigger!" She stomped out, swearing, and vowing to never return. In the exam room, her daughter-in-law exchanged hurried apologies and good-byes as Eleanor glared at us from across the waiting room.

I was surprised by Eleanor's language, by her inability to speak the word *dementia*, and by her anger. I was also grateful to be fired; there were other patients to see. I hurried to the physician workroom, dictated a summary of my encounter with Eleanor, and grabbed the next chart. I forgot about Eleanor.

But a month later, she showed up on my schedule again.

To my surprise, she was now resigned to my care. At her family's insistence, she had undergone the laboratory tests I recommended, and we reviewed them together. I told her that she was indeed experiencing dementia. I counseled her to give up the wine she enjoyed with dinner, sell her car, take an aspirin daily, and move to an assisted-living facility.

In the name of "harm-reduction," I was advising her to give up her independence, so I braced myself for more yelling. Instead, she obliged.

I was surprised but pleased, believing that Eleanor had, after a rough start, become the kind of algebra problem I desired. Simple.

But when she returned for a checkup months later, Eleanor brought an eight-page list of problems and one request: that we begin psychotherapy together. Instead of being an easily solved problem, she was going to demand my time. Years later, I realize that her demand taught me what it means to be seen by a physician, to trust a physician, and to hope in a physician; it also taught what I, as a physician, hope for while practicing medicine.

• • •

Since I first started seeing people as patients, I have been astounded by what they hope for when they visit physicians.

During my first week with the rural physician, when I saw Gloria die, the physician's office seemed to operate on a series of knowing winks. After each communication that sounded like a half-truth meant to appease a whining patient—the promise that the medications would help, that the cancer would remit, that life would be better—the physician would look my way and wink. When the physician was busy with the examination, a patient would look my way and wink at me while she told the physician how much she was drinking. After the lead nurse spoke disparagingly about one of the physician's assistants in the practice, she winked at me to signal it was our secret. Nobody even bothered to wink when the drug reps visited because, although they kept the office stocked with free drug samples and pens and notepads emblazoned with consonant-rich drug names that invoked health, they spoke in such baldly disingenuous terms that no one needed to feign sincerity in their presence. They did not rate a wink, but as the naive medical student performing his first digital rectal exam—"Sure, he's done this before. Now roll to the side, please"—I got winks from everyone involved as I lubed up.

The physician led the winking. People brought intractable problems to him with the same sort of unexplained need that leads well-fed house cats to kill birds and lay them before their masters. In Exam Room 1 was a middle-aged man who had lost his mother the previous year and whose wife had filed for divorce, and he wanted to know what the physician could do to help him. In Exam Room 2, a bewildered retiree reported a loss of energy and a floating sense of meaninglessness. In Exam Room 3, a meticulous woman presented the physician with a handwritten note asking why she often found lines on her feet after removing her socks and whether this was the sign of some Sunday-night-movie disease that would result in her dying, hair well-composed, during the third act. People carried their needs to the physician's office and then presented them one at a time, beginning with a backache and building to domestic abuse. They sought the kind of comfort contemporary medicine provides only despite itself, in the human interactions between physicians and patients, rather than in the drugs, co-payments, and insurance reimbursements explicitly exchanged in the office. So both parties winked a lot, trying to guide each other into the desired role. When it worked, patient and physician alike were exultant, as when the eighty-year-old woman was able to travel again after working out a new asthma regimen and brought the physician pictures of her trip, or when the thirty-five-year-old man was able to return to work and brought us out to the parking lot to show off the car he could now afford. When it failed, well, it was another alienating experience in an alienating culture, and patients returned home wondering why they had ever thought the physician would know what to do.

Many of the patients were beyond me, like the man in Exam Room 4 who had frontotemporal dementia that exhausted his wife. She still had all her faculties but could neither care for her husband nor give him up. In moments like that, all we could do was sit for a few minutes before moving on to the next exam room, with the hope that it would be occupied by someone we could help, someone we could shore up with drugs and regular office visits and winks. This was what constituted medical hope, I could tell. During my first two days in the clinic I performed two digital rectal exams, listened to the lungs of thirty patients, assisted in a pap smear, and gave a fifty-nine-year-old his yearly physical. His lungs sounded good, his heart sounded good, his ears looked good, his eyes looked good, his bowels sounded good, and his penis could still stand at attention when desire called its name. All good, I told him, and then winked to myself as I escorted him out of the exam room.

• • •

Six years later, working with Eleanor forced me to rethink what, beyond winking, physicians hope for.

When I met Eleanor, I was still trying to assume the identity of a psychiatrist—not the internist or surgeon I had initially planned to become. I was realizing that, at our best, psychiatrists help people live with their realities, but just like other physicians, psychiatrists often want to reduce patients to parts to be fixed and sources of income—parts and money. Where the money comes from varies more than for other physicians because of the vagaries of who does and does not have mental health insurance, but the part we need to fix seems obvious.

The brain.

We talk often about brain circuits and the messengers that traverse them. In this age of neuroscience, we are learning more every day. Among the advances that excite me are elegant experiments that show the brain's structure is not fixed in childhood, but changes in response to learning, which suggest that the brain can literally be altered through an experience like psychotherapy. I suspect that Jerome Frank would feel confirmed by these findings because he always believed that psychotherapy delivered in a therapeutic relationship could transform the meaning of an event. The Nobel Prize–winning psychiatrist Eric Kandel summarized these findings thus: "When a therapist speaks to a patient and the patient listens, the therapist is not only making eye contact and voice contact, but the action of neuronal machinery in the therapist's brain is having an indirect and, one hopes, long-lasting effect on the neuronal machinery in the patient's brain; and quite likely, vice versa."[1] In therapy, as patient and therapist examine and alter old ways of thinking and acting, they form new neuronal connections in their brains. Their brains actually change through the relationship they form. I appreciated this, so even though Eleanor's brain was shedding neuronal connections as her dementia progressed, my neuroscientific hope for her was that we could alter the "neuronal machinery" of her faltering brain, at least for a time, and that she could alter my own neuronal machinery in turn.

I shared some of these hopes with Eleanor, but I never told her about the other hopes that haunted me. I am, in the formulation of Walker Percy, a bad Catholic—someone who believes in God but does not see any reason why it should disturb his life.[2] I respect the lifework of Paul Farmer and Dorothy Day, Catholics who live in partnership with the poor, but I am hopelessly bourgeois. And I am no evangelist. I hesitate to discuss my faith with patients because I fear it would be coercive, and I do not know how to square psychiatry and Catholicism. The claim of psychiatry—in Freud's formulation, to restore patients to "common unhappiness"—is modest in comparison to the claim of the empty tomb.[3] I do not identify myself as a Catholic psychiatrist to patients, preferring to receive the assumptions they make on their own as evidence of how they think. But I do ask patients about their own faith and hopes.

When I asked Eleanor about these, she railed against the idea of hope, saying the world was so full of misery that any God must be so powerless as to be unworthy of belief. She said, "I hope in science. I hope in doctors. I want you to fix me." She wanted me to find her broken part, remove it or replace it, and send her back to her life.

I wanted to give Eleanor what she wanted.

• • •

People have mighty expectations of physicians and medicine.

I wanted to "fix" Eleanor, but what I could actually give her was a course of cognitive behavioral therapy (CBT), as a way of reducing her distress about being diagnosed with dementia. CBT is a newer psychotherapy whose efficacy has been demonstrated for multiple conditions. CBT researchers have generated an impressive body of evidence for its efficacy, even the kind of evidence Archie Cochrane described as the highest level. In CBT, a patient identifies unwanted behaviors and correlates them with distorted thinking by constructing "thought records," diagrams that reveal a patient's "core beliefs" about him- or herself and his or her relationships with other people.

I hoped CBT would help Eleanor accept her dementia, so we began with her angry response at being diagnosed with dementia, interpreting it as an "automatic thought" whose underlying "core belief" was a sense of helplessness. Eleanor saw that being unable to use words shamed her and reminded her of past experiences when she had been helpless and speechless. She recalled feeling speechless anger at her husband's repeated infidelities, but that wound was modest in comparison to her recollection of being to forced to masturbate the organist at her childhood church. She was perhaps five years old when it occurred, and she remembered helplessly trying to clean her dirtied hands. She had never told anyone, and she said she was relieved to finally tell me.

She connected those experiences with dementia, the loss of her words. She went on to learn breathing techniques to minimize her frustration over losing words. She developed memory aids to remember familiar people. Eleanor hoped that these gains would be enough, expressed satisfaction with her progress in CBT after twelve sessions, and fired me again.

CBT is designed to be a brief intervention, to end after about twelve sessions, so her decision was not unexpected. She had recognized that experiences of imposed silence induced feelings of helplessness, which led to anger and depression. She had learned new coping mechanisms. I thought she had reconciled herself to her diagnosis. I was pleased that we could relieve her distress in twelve sessions rather than years of therapy. I had fixed Eleanor's depression, solved for an x: an approximation of what Eleanor had asked for.

My enthusiasm at this conclusion now embarrasses me. How could I have thought that I could fix what was broken for Eleanor?

Three months later, Eleanor returned. She asked to resume psychotherapy but "without all that homework I hate and a chance to talk more about the past." Although Eleanor could identify benefits from CBT, she wanted to try psychoanalysis, an older psychotherapy that focuses on interpreting transference, the unresolved feelings a patient unconsciously redirects onto other people. Eleanor wanted to engage in a therapy that focuses on past experiences, especially from childhood, at precisely the time she was losing her memory.

This is decidedly not the hope of contemporary psychiatry, where psychoanalysis is a contested practice. Residents are still required to see patients in psychoanalysis, but they are often simultaneously hearing bitter testimonials from the faculty. Psychiatry training in the past usually required residents to undergo their own analysis, visiting a local analyst as often as five times a week for an hour of near-silent scrutiny of their unconscious, and then to submit their patients to the same. In my residency, most faculty members of earlier generations sharply contrasted the frustrations of psychoanalysis with the revelations of biological psychiatry, comparing biological psychiatry to a rural electricity project that illuminated the darkness of a scientific backwater.

Instead of speaking of id and ego, they wanted to talk about NMDA receptors and fMRI studies, to locate psychiatric distress in specific circuits of the brain rather than in an imagined topography of the psyche. We memorized Freud's defense mechanisms and schema of the unconscious for our yearly in-service exam, but otherwise the Viennese neurologist was simply the author of the unclaimed books sitting in our conference room with a sun-faded "free" sign in front of them. At one point, I realized that one of my fellow residents could not recognize Sigmund Freud in a picture. Psychiatrists are so focused on the brain, its neurotransmitters, and the drugs that modulate them that psychoanalysis is a marginalized practice. In a nod to that trend, another colleague in residency paid to have his first long white coat embroidered with the moniker "Brain Scientist."

Residents no longer undergo their own psychoanalysis as a matter of course, but they do see patients for psychodynamic therapy, a less intense version of psychoanalysis. Residents learn psychody-namic therapy through supervision with a master psychoanalyst to whom they apprentice. These psychoanalysts acknowledge that psy-choanalysis was once overused and inappropriate for many patients, but they insist that it remains a craft worth learning and a compelling way to engage patients one at a time.

My supervisor was David Moore. Before we met for the first time, I feared the expansiveness of psychoanalysis. The advantage of CBT, which is much more popular in contemporary psychiatry, is that it prizes efficient rationality, telling practitioners that unwanted behaviors are caused by distorted thinking and that if patients can change their thinking, they can change their associated behaviors. In CBT, just as in medical school, a patient could become someone else through study.

Psychoanalysis seemed to be a hermeneutics of the irrational. I worried that Eleanor and I would talk about sexual fantasies and bizarre dreams while ignoring her cognitive decline. My CBT su-pervisor had followed Eleanor's progress through rating scales that turned her depression and anxiety into a numerical score, an x we could solve, but Dr. Moore was not interested in rating scales. He wanted to me keep notes about how Eleanor dressed, sat, or gazed at me. Anything and everything was interpretable. He did not want me to take full responsibility for writing Eleanor's story, but to help her compose the next chapter.[4] He wanted me to listen well to Eleanor. In the face of my fears, I tried to borrow his imperturbable wisdom and pass it along to Eleanor.

When Eleanor and I met again in the clinic, we used a different room, and we used it in a different way. Instead of facing each other as we had in CBT, I sat at her side. I asked her to free-associate. In my notebook, I recorded her first response. She said, "You're a very important part of my life. I would not want anything to happen to anybody, especially to you." Suddenly, the transference, the unre-solved feelings from past relationships that she projected onto me, was apparent. She still struggled for words and names, but she now made associations she had not made in CBT. She imagined me as a lover, telling me, "I want to be treasured, to be loved, to steal you away." She connected life at her assisted-living facility with being a nurse in a British Army hospital: a regimented routine of meals and ministrations that nevertheless ended in death. She disliked the daily games of bingo and the forced cheerfulness of the place and felt that all the inhabitants were "being shaken down to the same kind of person they want us to be." She said that CBT felt comparable to this, like "a patch job to get me back onto a road which is still getting worse."

In the coming weeks, Eleanor reported that in therapy she could now be honest about her despair. She connected her shame at losing words with her sense that the universe itself was silent as she declined. She was raised an Anglican but considered herself an atheist. She could suppress or laugh at her decline for a time, but then she would say, "I have music, books, people, but something's missing. You wake up every morning, and it hits you again. Nothing's changed. I want what I can't have: a new life. I'm very angry with you, with my children, for keeping me here. If I was a believer, I would be angry at God."

She wanted to believe in something more than her own end, but she found the idea of God ridiculous in a world riven by violence. Death was her only future. She fantasized about an ideal suicide: a beach at sunset, a symphony orchestra, a bottle of wine, and a successful overdose. She was proud of her work as a nurse and proud of her children, but she despaired that she, like a guest who comes empty-handed to a potluck dinner, no longer had anything to give them. I suggested that our work itself might constitute a kind of hope, a way of making peace with the past. She shook off even this modest hope as a burden binding her to this life.

As we discussed the transference, Eleanor connected me to her father. In her dreams, she recalled the feeling of being safe at her father's side, the same side from which he occasionally asked her to dig out embedded shrapnel from combat wounds he suffered at Gallipoli. Eleanor experienced me as a man she could sit next to who was, like her father, not frightened by pain. She feared that I would leave her, just as her father did when he died in World War II, just as everyone upon whom she depended eventually did.

In the midst of our therapy, my wife became pregnant with our second child. Elin was a family medicine resident and planned to work until the day she delivered our daughter Mary Clare, take the available maternity time off, and then return to work. After Elin returned to work, I would stay home with our daughter for the three weeks of paternity leave the hospital allowed.

When I told Eleanor I would be taking paternity leave, she congratulated me, then she said, "You're a father, so I can't do that to you; I can't suicide." She wanted her suicide to be a private event, as unnoticed by the world as her dementia was unnoticed by God. She sometimes wished she had never had her own children because she felt unable to commit suicide without hurting them. She wanted no new friends because "they will only be someone else to mourn." Infants, children, and friends anchored Eleanor in this life, but she wanted out.

Eleanor fired me at the end of every session, even on the days when I thought we were making progress. I now suspected that firing me allowed her to act out her suicide, to be the one who decided when to leave.

As my paternity leave neared, Eleanor became more anxious. She began somaticizing, missing sessions because of headaches and nausea. She asked for permission to cry in an upcoming session, saying, "You know that soldiers' daughters don't cry." I had said this to her during our CBT course as a kind of summary of her core beliefs, of her stoicism, and Eleanor had thanked me for it often, calling it a balm. Now she finally wanted to cry. She wanted me to coax salty tears from her stony eyes.

When she returned the following week, she announced, "My eyes are so full of tears, but I just won't let them go." She asked for paper and a pen and then wrote, "Crying is for girls and silly women. No one can cry elegantly—I fight against it. You are too kind and pleasant so I have no target to dislike." She fired me again, then returned the next week for our scheduled appointment.

She said my impending paternity leave had altered our relationship because she could recognize that I was a kind of parent to her, a parent who would be absent in her time of need. Her father had died in combat while Eleanor was on the home front nursing. When she returned from the front, she nursed her mother through terminal cancer of the bone. As we discussed the implications of my own leave, she finally discussed her mother: "When you had a stomachache, she got brown paper, ironed it, and placed it on your tummy. It felt so good. That's the hardest thing to lose, the warm place. When I would go to sleep, she would say, 'If you are frightened in the night, remember that I am holding your hand.' That was an astonishingly strong belief, that she was holding my hand in the night. . . . She can't hold my hand anymore. That's why there is no God in my brain anymore. No one should have been crucified like she was. If there is a God, I can't believe in Him."

Thinking of her mother, she paused and then said, "I just want to be suckled down to the grave." I was awed by her candor, by her raw expression of need. My imminent paternity leave was changing the transference, the unresolved feelings that Eleanor projected onto me. I was now a kind of mother, and she was more ambivalent than ever about therapy. She would now begin sessions by saying, "I'm coming to you to see how you feel about me quitting" and then, moments later, "I don't want to quit, in fact, I never want to leave." Eleanor needed other people—her children, her mother, the staff at her facility, me—but felt ashamed by her need.

I once saw her looking mournfully at the clock that hung in our therapy room, the clock that measured out our halting conversations. When I asked why she was sad, she said, "I'm scared of that clock because it goes fast and when it goes, you're gone."

The clock was moving too fast for Eleanor because time was running out on her sessions, therapy, cognitive ability, and life. Eleanor was slipping into a wordless dementia that prefigured what she understood death to be, a silent grave. Eleanor invited me to look at this dark earth every time we met. I looked with her, but I also asked if there were another vista. She said no. She could imagine no ascent, no hope beyond the grave.

Was Eleanor right? Was her hopelessness a symptom of her depression, a sober accounting of what she was losing to dementia, or the unhappy result of facing the finitude of life? She often told me, "There is no God," but she asked me several times if I believed in one. I played by the psychoanalytic rules and parried the question. She would nod at my deflections and then address the same question obliquely, again expressing her ambivalence about being dependent upon other people.

"I don't feel connected to anything—all my kids, you, doing things for me, I just feel I'm, I can't think of the word, where there is nothing."

"Death?"

"I don't think so, but that would make sense."

"Dementia?"

"Well, I asked you and you said it. I'm not sure I like that answer. I could trip over the kettle with that word. I didn't think I had anything left to lose. I had already lost writing, painting, speaking, a lot of things. I want the loss to stop. I think you should change the name of the illness to 'hope.'"

I was struck by her non-sequitur, perhaps produced by her difficulty with word finding, but incisive all the same. She had stated the question of her psychotherapy: How do you change dementia into hope? I tried to help her imagine, if not the ascending hope of a hymn, something more approachable. When she complained about how small she felt when she needed the assistance of her son to attend appointments or remember dates, I asked if he had learned to walk or talk on his own, reminding her that others had once depended upon her.

While I was home on paternity leave, I thought about Eleanor often. Was I prolonging Eleanor's torment by seeking hope?

When I returned, Eleanor and I had few opportunities to answer these questions. She cancelled several appointments. When we did meet, she seemed more confused than before. She continued to struggle with word finding and memory loss, but mostly with her growing dependence on other people for every activity.

Now she fired me two or three times a session. I no longer wanted to be fired; indeed, I looked forward to our conversations as a respite. Working with Eleanor, being present to her in her suffering without worrying about fixing a broken part or generating money, felt like being a real physician.

When Eleanor and I did meet, I continued to seek other hopes, asking if her own death could be a kind of extension of her work as a hospice nurse, of teaching others how to die. She despaired, saying, "I know what you're saying and I appreciate it, but it's just such a waste. There's nothing there—if you take a can opener and open my brain, there's nothing there and I resent that. It's in the cold, dark moments of the night, well, there's the dying right there." After this comment, this statement of how little she could hope for with a brain that was missing the words and names and memories that constituted her very self, I had the borrowed sense to be silent.

We met once more. In the middle of our final session, she abruptly addressed her lack of faith.

"I'm supposed to go to God, I think."

"Did I ask about God? What brought God to your mind?"

"You didn't bring it up, but I want to know what will happen. As far as God is concerned, if He is that powerful, why do all these terrible things happen? I think He's just a liar. How much would it have cost Him to save my mother from cancer?"

Eleanor was asking questions of theodicy, questions for which psychiatry had no answer. In my notebook, the last words I recorded from Eleanor are "I want to vanish. I know I've got to live until I die. It's not what I want, but it's what I have, it's what I have." She missed her next appointment. The following week, her son called and told me that his mother had decided to end therapy. Three years after we met, Eleanor had fired me for the last time.

I was devastated. What did Eleanor's silence mean?

Her absence left me with questions about what I came to regard as a physician's hope, something decidedly more modest than the hope of the neuroscientist and the hope of the saint, but the same hope Eleanor had offered her mother, the wounded soldiers she cared for, her children, and her hospice patients: the hope of having company in the face of implacable loss.

Eleanor imagined me as a technician, a father, a lover, a mother. I could be none of the things, but I could allow her to imagine.

And who did I imagine I was when I was with Eleanor?

I started out as burned-out resident, hoping she would miss her appointment.

When she did show up, I tried to be the author who gathered the seemingly disparate strands of her story into a single compelling narrative, a story called dementia. The story was accurate, but it was a medical story, not Eleanor's story. I saw pathology, a broken part, and while I was correct in my diagnosis, I wonder whether I did her a disservice. My diagnosis led directly to her giving up wine, which she loved, and to her moving to a nursing home, which she hated. By naming her "demented," I left her diminished.

I tried to be her technician, working through her anxious and depressed thoughts about being diagnosed with dementia. We used an evidence-based manual. We followed it scrupulously. We assessed her responses using standardized scales. And yet we had never addressed the meaning of her dementia and her eventual death.

When we finally addressed their significance, I offered her my time and attention in a way that was distinct from how I usually engaged with a patient. I became a kind of servant to her. Instead of offering a diagnosis or medicine, I offered myself as an aid to her health. Our work was halting, and I stumbled along the way, but being a kind of servant was the best I could do.

Afterward, I went back to the clinic's discard pile and read one of Freud's books. Much of it seemed better as literary criticism than as medical advice, but it was shot through with moments of wisdom, such as when he advised physicians who practice psychoanalysis to remember the motto of the Renaissance surgeon Ambroise Paré: "Je le pansai, Dieu le guérit" (I dressed his wounds, God cured him).[5]

What would it have been like to live in a world like Paré's, where people shared at least some mutual hope in God, in ultimate things, in a sense of what happens after our death? Eleanor and I did not share such hopes. Physicians and patients rarely do today. So what can we do? How can we go on together? The consensus of Ambroise Paré's time seems unlikely to return.

But what we can do is think of ourselves as something more than technicians in control of the body. At times, we can be like gardeners, teachers, servants, or witnesses to the people we meet as patients. Six years into medical practice, I feel as though my search for wisdom has just begun, but I know these models are all part of the finest traditions of my calling. They all share a humbler sense of who a physician is, a more limited sense of a physician's responsibility for the meaning of a patient's life, and a language to describe, out of the faint shadows, what makes medical practice still worthwhile.

There is another role for a physician that also makes medical practice worthwhile, that of ship's captain.

• • •

Every morning when I rise, I gaze upon an image of Basil of Caesarea, the man who founded the first public hospital. In the image, Basil is holding an unfurled scroll upon which an excerpt from his rules for living, an ancient version of a checklist, is written.

In his rules, Basil endorsed the practice of medicine so long as the patient and physician understood what they were getting into. He enumerated the benefits of being under the care of a physician and receiving the "cutting, burning, and the taking of bitter medicines for the cure of the body"—the evidence-based recommendations of his era. He criticized the misuse of medicine, describing it as an "outrage" and wrote, "To place the hope of one's health in the hands of the doctor is the act of an irrational animal. This, nevertheless, is what we observe in the case of certain unhappy persons who do not hesitate to call their doctors their saviors."[6] Every morning, when

I read Basil's reminders, I think about how medicine can help the patients I will see that day and how it can hurt them. Every morning, I remember again that when we place our hope in physicians, we become irrational animals because we expect physicians to save us from the decline and death that is our common lot.

Basil insisted that we should neither place our hope in medicine nor repudiate its gifts. Instead, he wrote, "As we entrust the helm to the pilot in the art of navigation, but implore God that we may end our voyage unharmed by the perils of the sea, so also, when reason allows, we call in the doctor, but we do not leave off hoping in God."[7]

Some mornings, I think about Eleanor while looking at the image of Basil. Eleanor both trusted me and placed hope in me, but Basil distinguished between trusting and placing hope in physicians. For Basil, the ship's captain commanded the ship but not his passengers. When you board a ship, you trust the captain to take you safely to your destination. When you disembark, you trust in other people; no one asks the captain how to navigate life ashore. The relationship with the captain is temporary, its scope limited to a particular journey. You trust the captain to transport you safely, but you do not place hope in the captain for something outside of his navigational duties.

Illness is not algebra, but a journey into dark waters. When you are ill, you need a captain, and I take Basil to mean that a physician can be our captain during an illness without taking authority for our lives outside of that illness. If physicians are this kind of captain, we can trust their expertise during specific times of need without allowing them control over our bodies and lives. Physicians who understand themselves as this kind of captain would acknowledge that as death nears their role recedes. Instead of spending our last moments being examined by teams of physicians, residents, and students, we might thank the physician-captain for his or her assistance and turn to others for help with death. We could trust physicians to diagnose illnesses, prescribe treatments, and respond to complications, but we would finally trust other people to decide the meaning of our bodies and lives. Might that be a relief to patient and physician alike? After all, whatever comes after this life, there is no medical destination.

Imagining physicians as more like captains encourages patients to place their hope elsewhere while relieving physicians of a burdensome responsibility. That seems like the true ground for the renewal of medicine. So when I enter the hospital every morning, a structure inspired by Basil's commitment to care for the indigent stranger and Osler's commitment to seeing much, I try to see each patient, however obscured by his or her infirmities and vulnerabilities, as a person.

• • •

When I enter our gleaming hospital buildings, my journey has taught me that they may be physically beautiful, but they are, even by their own accounts, ineffective and inefficient. And yet I still work in one of these buildings every day. Like most physicians, I have many roles at the hospital. Looking over my appointments from the past week, I see meetings where I worked as a clinician, a teacher, a researcher, an administrator, a quality-improvement officer, an electronic medical record builder, and an agent of the state. Each role has attendant skills and responsibilities. Each role has its time and place. But I fear that the personal roles are being deemphasized in favor of the population-based roles. In residency, I trained in the craft of psychotherapy, but the healthcare industry discouraged me from practicing therapy. I am encouraged to engage in the activities that only a physician can undertake, which usually means diagnosing complex cases, prescribing medications, and designing the algorithms of evidence-based and standardized care rather than sitting with people like Eleanor for an hour every week. When we speak of fixing and reforming healthcare, it is primarily by encouraging roles that discourage physicians from engaging patients as individuals. We encourage physicians to see a patient as a representative of a population group rather than as a particular person shaped by his or her particular communities and experiences.

In short, we call for physicians to see much.

We need to see wisely. After all, the opportunity of medicine is that you meet people every day who are quite different from yourself, and they grant you an opportunity to see them well by serving them in their suffering. Each person is particular and can only be known through a relationship formed in a particular place and time. After witnessing so many reform initiatives sweep through the hospital, I hope we can renew medicine on an individual basis—not through a big, top-down reform—in which we form therapeutic alliances to help patients achieve something they could not achieve on their own and witness the hardships they experience. The solution for medicine's ails is not rigid standardization but the renewal of wisdom and the communities that cultivate wisdom. The renewal of medicine begins by opening cultural spaces for local, particular communities where people can meet together like the irrational animals that we are.

Eleanor gave me that hope.

He spoke in an improvised rhythm, starting out fast, flying up the register, skittering from bright thought to bright thought. I struggled to follow his lines, so I asked him to slow up, to talk along with me, so that I could appreciate the forces at work in his mind. Now he repeated words, using his sculpted lips and tapered hands, to tell me about the voices, voices, voices. "They come at night, night, night and tell me to die, die, die. All right, all right, all right. Tip-tap, tip-tap, tip-tap." He moved his feet in time with his voice and then accelerated his speech again. As he ascended into the crazed rhythm of clang associations, he shone like the saxophone he played with those hands and those lips.

I could have listened to Gregorio all day.

Unlike many of the people I meet on the psychiatric ward, Gregorio shone. I mean his pants were clean, his shirt creased, and his hair newly cut—strange enough on our ward—but also that he seemed to emit a warm light. He was the kind of man that women would want to sit next to on the bus. Most of the people I meet on the ward are the kind whom you would avoid whether on a bus or in a bar, even if it meant having to stand. They are usually poor and imperiled by their illness. They take orders from unseen forces, tune into stations in their heads that no one else can hear, and frighten people in bars and on buses. Sometimes, they frighten me.

On paper, Gregorio sounded like one of those people. He had been hospitalized because voices were telling him to kill himself, a common refrain on the ward. Like many of the young men I meet, Gregorio had begun life sweetly enough, with an occasional sour melody that was at first an interruption, but that eventually became an incessant refrain. He was raised by a single mother. He enlisted in the army to pay for a bachelor's degree in music but left the service because he disliked violence. He toured as a saxophonist and then began an MBA to figure out how to turn gigs into a career. But the voices intervened.

He had been kicked off his last tour, hospitalized in a distant city, and then discharged to the Greyhound station. He was sent back home to live in his mother's basement. After six months of that—doing okay, playing along—he suffered more loss, the murder of a brother, the suicide of a girlfriend: the dissonant chords of being black, poor, and mentally ill in a society that stigmatized all three.

So his mother cared for him—her favorite son, her youngest, her only living child—but she brought him to the hospital when the voices persisted, hoping to shelter him more safely there. She knew what the voices meant. Schizophrenia ran through the family. It had taken her father, her oldest son, and now Gregorio. Schizophrenia, with its fainter hammers to the head, had become her family's full music.

At the Psychiatric Emergency Department, it is never night, but never dawn either. The lights are fluorescent, the windows are bricked-in, and the clocks face the staff. All you see are the nurses. They sit behind security glass, reinforced with a lattice of steel mesh. Sometimes a nurse comes out from behind the glass. She asks questions. Checks your temperature. Draws blood. Collects urine. Food comes. Time slips. The physician sees you. You try to explain inner voices and outer voices to him. He tells you that you will be hospitalized.

When there is a bed, you come upstairs to the ward. We have windows. We have sunlight. We have a clock you can see. The day's schedule is clearly posted.

On the schedule, it says physicians make rounds in the morning between 7 and 11. I make those rounds to see patients who, like Gregorio, are hospitalized against their will because someone decided they are mentally ill and a danger to themselves or others. These are potent phrases, but also euphemisms. What do we mean by mental illness, by danger?

Mental illness is a social construct, a divine curse, a neurobiological illness.

Danger is a schoolyard slur, a drunken threat, a determined act.

My job is to define these vague terms for each patient, to sift out the mentally ill from the malingerers, the truly damaged from the ordinary wounded, and the imminently dangerous from those who will explode only under particular pressures. To do so, I ask a lot of questions, but I often forget that these questions, while informative, can be more intrusive than illuminating. Gregorio is a reminder of the difference.

I learned much from Eleanor, but she was the last patient I saw in psychotherapy. The notebooks in which I transcribed our encounters now sit inside my desk in the back hallway of a locked psychiatric unit. I practice in one of Basil's hospitals rather than one of Freud's clinics.

When I finished residency, I wanted to work at Denver Health because it allowed me to be a kind of servant in my home state. I had gone away for training, but I wanted my children to know their grandparents, aunts, and uncles, and to grow up alongside their cousins. One of the great privileges of being a physician—and there are many—is that I could choose where to work. I am privileged to work here, a place where I can be a physician to indigent ill people like Gregorio.

Working here, I often move among roles. When I fit Gregorio's experiences into a diagnostic criteria set, I act as an author of Gregorio, the patient. When I select a treatment for him after reviewing the available scientific evidence, I am an epidemiologist. When I follow standardized checklists to ensure he receives evidence-based care, I am a technician. When I help him achieve a level of health he could not achieve on his own, I am a coach. When I teach him about his illness and its treatments, I am a teacher. When I ask about the people and places in his life and how they affect his health, I am a gardener. When I return at the day's end to sit with and listen to him, I am a servant. When I tell other people about the many ways we fail Gregorio, I am a witness. When I help him with all his medical needs without taking full responsibility for his successes or failures, I am like a ship's captain. Throughout, I am privileged to attend to Gregorio.

In these roles, I see Gregorio in different ways. At times, he is a source of income. I am no doctor without silver, but a salaried employee of Denver Health. Being a salaried employee frees me from many incentives to overtest and overtreat patients, but it also means I cannot operate a private practice on the side, as physicians in a previous generation did, the kind of private practice where I could see patients like Eleanor. I miss that lost opportunity, but the salary is regular and allows me to keep pace with my student loans and to support my family.

At other times, I see Gregorio as a collection of parts. I am fascinated by neuroscience, by the circuits and neurotransmitters that are operating within Gregorio's brain when we sit together. I am amazed by remarkable pathologies and frightening derangements. I find myself swapping stories with colleagues, then feeling embarrassed because my own health, in comparison, is good. It is much easier to be a physician than a patient.

But someday I will, of course, be the patient. That time comes for us all. I worry about what kind of physicians I will encounter. Every few months, a new version of healthcare reform whips through the hospital, as constantly changing as the weather. Some people argue that paying physicians for performance and outcomes is real reform. Performance and outcomes are important, but they are no more than a standardized and scaled version of the view of patients as parts and money. I suspect that real reform will come only when we change what physicians and other practitioners see in the people they meet as patients, and when we allow patients to see us in return.

I want to tell you what Gregorio saw in me.

I met Gregorio for the first time the morning after his mother brought him to the hospital. Whereas I had slept at home in my own bed, he had slept on a molded polymer bed bolted to the floor of the Psychiatric Emergency Department. After telling her son's story in the Emergency Department, his mother had gone home, where she could sleep, for the first time in months, without checking on him every half-hour. In her absence, Gregorio became upset. The psychiatric emergency nurses tried to reason with him, but he was beyond their reason. Eventually, they used Velcro to affix his wrists and ankles to the plastic bed that was bolted to the floor of the windowless room, and they induced sleep with "10 and 2," hospital slang for 10 milligrams of haloperidol and 2 milligrams of lorazepam, sedating doses of medications administered intramuscularly.

I read all this information at the nurses' station on our ward, where I stop in each morning to review the records of the patients admitted overnight. After receiving his meds, Gregorio had been sent upstairs at four in the morning. When he arrived, the ward nurses could not get much out of him. Since he could no longer speak for himself, they described him. "Isolated. Calmed." More euphemisms.

I let Gregorio continue sleeping while I saw other patients. Later in the morning, I found a room and a few chairs. I woke Gregorio and asked him to join me. We sat together and he told his story.

"My mother knows I've been under a lot of stress, stress, stress. I dropped out of school, school, school. I didn't get the help I needed, so I hear voices, voices, voices. I want them to stop, stop, stop." His words were staccato but clear.

My own hands and lips cannot play any instrument, but I have learned to follow along with people like Gregorio. They sing, they stutter, and I keep time with them, trying to discern why, why, why they are ill enough to be hospitalized. Every song is distinct, but I have learned how to accompany each player. Sometimes I summarize, sometimes I redirect, and sometimes I just listen.

When I started out as a student, I found these rhythms unintelligible, so I asked questions that made sense to me, mostly questions on the hospital forms I was completing. "What is your chief complaint? How would you describe your mood? Do you see things other people do not see?" My questions were informative for me, but not for my patients. They presented with personal concerns, and I responded with questions from a preprinted list of symptoms.

Fifteen years later, I find myself asking someone else to sing the tune so I can follow along. I start by asking people what they like to be called. I listen. I ask, "Why do you believe you are ill?" When I asked Gregorio this, he began to cry, then fell mute. After a few minutes, he said, "I cannot tell anyone, but maybe you . . . " He straightened his index finger and pointed at the hospital-issued identification badge that hung around my neck. My picture is on the badge, with my expanding forehead and the same tentative smile I offered to assistant principals who discovered me reading novels under the stairwell when I should have been in gym class.

As he pointed, Gregorio said, "The nerds. The nerds. The nerds have lost their luster."

"Are you pointing at my badge because you see me as a nerd?" He nodded, looked up, and smiled. "Like you? Are we both nerds?" He nodded again, smiled again, and now we could talk. We talked about old records, obscure movies, and out-of-print books. The nerds were shining together. Skipping gym class together.

The languages of medicine are German and Greek, and they reflect our sense that health is an adherence to an ideal form and illness is a deviation. So when physicians account for our patients, we use terms that outline the geographies of these ideal forms. In psychiatry, the geographies can be imagined (id, ego, superego) or structural (amygdala, hippocampus, thalamus), but they are often descriptive. We describe a patient's speech as slowed or rapid, alliterative or accented, aphonic or mute. We describe his or her affect as stable or labile, as restricted or constricted, euphoric or dysphoric. We describe the patient's thought process as organized or derailed, logical or illogical, intact or circumstantial. Assign enough descriptions, and they assemble into a diagnosis.

The psychiatrist Paul McHugh charges that we have become birders, comparing people to our handbooks and determining their illness based on their external characteristics.[1] Delusions? Hallucinations? Disorganized speech? Lasting at least six months? Must be schizophrenia.

As a word, *schizophrenia* sounds Greek, but it was introduced into the language by a psychiatrist lecturing in 1908.[2] The name has little music to it. The five syllables that make up *schizophrenia* are of varying length. Two long Greek roots, "to split" and "mind," bound together around that harsh *o*. The word is misused all the time. Psychiatrists dislike hearing it used to mean "of two minds" or "having multiple personalities." The word was created by one of our own, and we claim the authority to use it.

But we have our own misuses of the word. We give it to other people as a name—they do not so much have schizophrenia as they become a schizophrenic. From there, it is easy to become a "schiz-o" a dulling name for a person.

Psychiatrists lament the stigmatization experienced by our patients, the way they are caricatured as dangerous, dim-witted, or dull. And yet our diagnostic system makes little room for the particular passions of a person. Our encounters focus on pathologies rather than strengths, and our language has no account for a man who, while he hears frightening voices, still shines.

Luster enters English from the French *lustre*, the Italian *lustro*, and the Latin *lustrare*. All the Romance words end with a vowel, with a sound that invites the lips to expand and the mind to alight upon some of its meanings: a reflected glory, a polished shine, an illuminating light.

That first night after I met him, I thought about Gregorio. How, exactly, did the nerds lose their luster? When engineers make billions as entrepreneurs, can the nerds possibly have any more luster?

I was a bookish boy and capitalized on my habits to become a physician. Gregorio was a bookish boy as well, but what had happened to his share of luster? I still do not know why some have many chances to shine and some have very few—these are questions for theodicy not psychiatry—but I know that I awoke the next day eager to speak with Gregorio.

At the hospital, the overnight notes indicated he had done well. I thought we would pick up where we left off the day before. Instead, when I approached him on the ward, he was shaking. Unbidden, my mind formulated a differential diagnosis—anxiety, withdrawal, adverse med effects—and I thought like a physician: "What part is broken?" We physicians think so much about broken parts that when we see something out of the ordinary, we immediately seek the fault, naming it with our distancing, dulling language. Was Gregorio anxious because of impaired activity in his amygdala, undisclosed alcohol dependence, or akathisia from excessive dopamine blockade?

I was trying to locate Gregorio's experience on one of our geographies, when I saw what he was holding in his tremulous hands: stock reports. He was carrying the annual reports of Fortune 500 companies. I asked why he carried them. His eyes welled with tears as he slowly handed me a glossy report, its cardstock pages fluttering in the air-conditioned breeze. I read the words on its cover—*We've Got You Under Our Wing: Annual Report, Aflac Incorporated.* A cartoon duck's sheltering wings were spread out in invitation.

"Is that for me?"

Gregorio nodded.

"Why?"

He stammered, "I, I, I have been thinking you. I wanted to make sure that you were covered, that if anything happened to you, you could stay home, sit in your psychiatrist chair, and be safe."

Usually, when patients say they have been thinking about me, they mean they have been thinking about how they will convince me to discharge them. Gregorio was thinking about the possibility that I might someday be ill or injured and need supplemental insurance. He was thinking about me as a person who could suffer. I was astounded.

Is the empathy of his prisoners too much for a jailer to ask?

I do not like to think of myself as a jailer, but that is how many of my patients conceive of me. After all, when society grants me the authority to define dangerousness and mental illness, it also grants me the authority to restrict the freedoms of the people I meet as patients. With the right words on the right form, I can hold a person, against his or her will, in our hospital for days, weeks, or even months. Under extreme circumstances, I can administer involuntary medications. "Please take this pill. If you do not, the nurses will have to inject you with these medicines." My tongue has become accustomed to the language of coercion, with its careful phrases and its cloaked threats, followed by the nurses counting off one-two-three fingerbreadths below the shoulder's bony acromion so they can sink the needle into the deltoid.

Gregorio was using a different language, the language of personal concern. Within a few days, he would still be hearing voices, but he would be able to talk back to them. He was engaged in treatment. He was making plans for the future. He was going to see a psychiatrist when he left. He was going to live with his mother again. He was thinking about other people.

This is a rare thing on the ward. A colleague of mine is legally blind. She wears glasses so powerful that her pupils appear twice as large as their actual size. She has worked on the ward for almost thirty years, but she has told me that only once, in all those years, did a patient pull out a chair for her. She was touched by his kindness, by his ability to perceive her impairment and to assist her. She says it is more typical for patients who observe her impairment to blurt out something rude. She knows this is often a symptom of the conditions our patients experience, that they forget how to interact with other people, so she no longer takes it personally. She chooses to take only the kindnesses personally. She remembers the gentleman who pulled out her chair.

I remember Gregorio.

After forming an alliance with Gregorio, we could listen to each other, and offer a warm concern for each other as fellow creatures. I could see that his concern for other people was the source of his luster. I could also see that sharing a bit of the luster of people like Gregorio is how we physicians will endure in medicine, even as healthcare reforms. Sitting with Gregorio I see that what passes for healthcare reform is variations on parts and money, with promises to hospitals, insurers, pharmaceutical manufacturers, and, yes, physicians, that their profits are assured. Sitting with Gregorio generates little income and requires me to think about him as something more than his parts. Sitting with Gregorio, searching for luster, is the grounds for the renewal of medicine. So I have learned to tinker with the various systems designed to optimize the treatment of parts and collection of money. I find cracks and crevices in the day where I can sit with a patient like Gregorio and attempt to see that patient as an individual and, on the best occasions, to be seen in turn by him or her. I feel often like the protagonist of Walker Percy's novel *The Moviegoer*, who concludes "There is only one thing I can do: listen to people, see how they stick themselves into the world, hand them along a ways in their dark journey and be handed along, and for good and selfish reasons."[3] Percy was a physician. I imagine he would have liked Gregorio.

I know I did, because on that day, Gregorio saw me. In the midst of our dark journeys, we handed each other along, and I experienced the joy of healing someone who sought my help.

He returned a month later. He asked to see me. He wanted to give his card to the nerd.

I keep it on my desk. It is the standard size, a rectangle 3 1/2 by 2 inches, but it is oriented vertically, unlike most business cards. In the upper-right-hand corner is his name, followed by his occupation and phone number. In the lower-right-hand corner there is a picture of Gregorio, his lips pursed, preparing to blast straight 8s and push the rhythm.

I can only hope to keep up with those who, like Gregorio, seek my help.

NOTES

Introduction

1. This account follows from Michel Foucault, *The Birth of the Clinic: An Archaeology of Medical Perception*, trans. A. M. Sheridan (New York: Pantheon, 1973).

2. See Tait D. Shanafelt, Sonja Boone, Litjen Tan, Lotte N. Dyrbye, et al., "Burnout and Satisfaction with Work-Life Balance Among US Physicians Relative to the General US Population." *Archives of Internal Medicine* 172, no. 18 (2012): 1377–85.

Chapter 1. Seeing Wisely

1. Abraham Flexner and Carnegie Foundation for the Advancement of Teaching, *Medical Education in the United States and Canada: A Report to the Carnegie Foundation for the Advancement of Teaching* (New York: Carnegie Foundation for the Advancement of Teaching, 1910).

2. Osler delivered the speech in 1894, and it was later disseminated in a collection of his writings. See William Osler, "The Army Surgeon," in *Aequanimitas*, 2nd ed. (Philadelphia: P. Blakinson's Son, 1914), 105–20.

3. Sylvio LeBlond, "The Life and Times of Alexis St-Martin," *Canadian Medical Association Journal* 88 (1963): 1205–11.

4. Osler, "Army Surgeon," 120.

5. Osler's essay was published in William Beaumont and William Osler, *Experiments and Observations on the Gastric Juice and the Physiology of Digestion Together with a Biographical Essay, "William Beaumont: A Pioneer American Physiologist"* (Mineola, N.Y.: Dover, 1996). The best overview of Osler's life is Michael Bliss, *William Osler: A Life in Medicine* (New York: Oxford University Press, 1999). The characterization of "old fistulous Alexis," comes from LeBlond, "Life and Times of Alexis St-Martin," 1209.

6. For example, see Howard Markel, "Experiments and Observations: How William Beaumont and Alexis St. Martin Seized the Moment of Scientific Progress." *JAMA* 302, no. 7 (2009): 804–6.

7. R. L. Golden, "Sir William Osler and the Anatomical Tubercle," *Journal of the American Academy of Dermatology* 16, no. 5, pt. 1 (1987): 1071–74.
8. James R. Wright, "Sins of Our Fathers: Two of the Four Doctors and Their Roles in the Development of Techniques to Permit Covert Autopsies," *Archives of Pathology and Laboratory Medicine* 133, no. 12 (2009): 1969–74.
9. George S. M. Dyer and Mary E. L. Thorndike, "Quidne mortui vivos docent? The Evolving Purpose of Human Dissection in Medical Education," *Academic Medicine* 75, no. 10 (2000): 969–79.
10. Michel Foucault, *The Birth of the Clinic: An Archaeology of Medical Perception*, trans. A. M. Sheridan (New York: Pantheon, 1973), 146.

Chapter 2. Occult Findings

1. Osler delivered the speech, "Internal Medicine as a Vocation," in 1897, but it was disseminated in *Aequanimitas*, 2nd ed. (Philadelphia: P. Blakinson's Son, 1914), 139–152, quotation on p. 144.
2. Alvin E. Rodin, "Osler's Autopsies: Their Nature and Utilization." *Medical History* 17, no. 1 (1973): 37–48.
3. Abraham Flexner and Carnegie Foundation for the Advancement of Teaching, *Medical Education in the United States and Canada: A Report to the Carnegie Foundation for the Advancement of Teaching* (New York: Carnegie Foundation for the Advancement of Teaching, 1910), 95, 68; Walter E. Finkbeiner, Philip C. Ursell, and Richard L. Davis, *Autopsy Pathology: A Manual and Atlas*, 2nd ed. (Philadelphia: Saunders/Elsevier, 2009), 8.
4. See Finkbeiner, Ursell, and Davis, *Autopsy Pathology*.
5. Quoted in Michel Foucault, *The Birth of the Clinic: An Archaeology of Medical Perception*, trans. A. M. Sheridan (New York: Pantheon, 1973), 146.
6. Foucault, *Birth of the Clinic*, 146.

Chapter 3. The Book and the Coat

1. Dan W. Blumhagen, "The Doctor's White Coat: The Image of the Physician in Modern America," *Annals of Internal Medicine* 91, no. 1 (1979): 111–16.
2. C. Stewart Rogers, "UNC White Coat Ceremony: Keynote Address 2000," *Forum of the North Carolina Medical Board* 5, no. 4 (2000): 5–6.

3. Arnold Gold and Sandra Gold, "Humanism in Medicine from the Perspective of the Arnold Gold Foundation: Challenges to Maintaining the Care in Health Care," *Journal of Child Neurology* 21, no. 6 (2006): 546.

4. Gold and Gold, "Humanism in Medicine from the Perspective of the Arnold Gold Foundation," 547.

5. See, for example, Judah L. Goldberg, "Humanism or Professionalism? The White Coat Ceremony and Medical Education," *Academic Medicine* 83, no. 8 (2008): 715–22; Philip C. Russell. "The White Coat Ceremony: Turning Trust into Entitlement," *Teaching and Learning in Medicine* 14, no. 1 (2002): 56–59; Robert M. Veatch, "White Coat Ceremonies: A Second Opinion," *Journal of Medical Ethics* 28, no. 1 (2002): 5–9; and Delese Wear, "On White Coats and Professional Development: The Formal and the Hidden Curricula," *Annals of Internal Medicine* 129, no. 9 (1998): 734–37.

6. Gold and Gold, "Humanism in Medicine from the Perspective of the Arnold Gold Foundation," 546.

7. Moses Maimonides, "Oath of Maimonides," trans. Harry Friedenwald, *Bulletin of Johns Hopkins Hospital* 28 (1917): 260–61.

8. Ryan M. Antiel, Farr A. Curlin, C. Christopher Hook, and Jon C. Tilburt, "The Impact of Medical School Oaths and Other Professional Codes of Ethics: Results of a National Physician Survey," *Archives of Internal Medicine* 171, no. 5 (2011): 469–71.

9. T. Jock Murray, "Read Any Good Books Lately?" *McGill Journal of Medicine* 12, no. 1 (2009): 90–91.

10. John Stone and Richard C. Reynolds, "*On Doctoring:* The Making of an Anthology of Literature and Medicine," in *To Improve Health and Health Care: The Robert Wood Johnson Foundation Anthology* (San Francisco: Jossey-Bass, 2003).

11. William Osler, "The Army Surgeon," in *Aequanimitas*, 2nd ed. (Philadelphia: P. Blakinson's Son, 1914), 104.

12. William Osler, "Books and Men," in *Aequanimitas*, 220.

Chapter 4. Full Responsibility

1. Abraham Verghese, *My Own Country: A Doctor's Story of a Town and Its People in the Age of AIDS* (New York: Simon and Schuster, 1994), 263. (My quotations are taken from the original hardcover edition, cited here; the paperback, published by Vintage, is subtitled simply "A Doctor's Story.")

2. Verghese, *My Own Country*, 25.
3. Verghese, *My Own Country*, 319.
4. Abraham Verghese, "The Physician as Storyteller," *Annals of Internal Medicine* 135, no. 11 (2001): 1016.
5. Verghese, *My Own Country*, 342.
6. Jeffrey P. Bishop, "Rejecting Medical Humanism: Medical Humanities and the Metaphysics of Medicine," *Journal of Medical Humanities* 29, no. 1 (2008): 16.
7. Richard T. Penson, Lidia Schapira, Sally Mack, Marjorie Stanzler, and Thomas J. Lynch, "Connection: Schwartz Center Rounds at Massachusetts General Hospital Cancer Center," *Oncologist* 15, no. 7 (2010): 762.
8. Penson et al., "Connection," 760.

Chapter 5. Duty Hours

1. ABIM Foundation, American Board of Internal Medicine, ACP-ASIM Foundation, American College of Physicians—American Society of Internal Medicine, and European Federation of Internal Medicine, "Medical Professionalism in the New Millennium: A Physician Charter," *Annals of Internal Medicine* 136, no. 3 (2002): 243–46.
2. Marjorie Lehman O'Rorke, North Carolina Office of Archives and History, and North Carolina Department of Cultural Resources, *Haven on the Hill: A History of North Carolina's Dorothea Dix Hospital* (Raleigh: Office of Archives and History, North Carolina Dept. of Cultural Resources, 2010). I also consulted the history page maintained by the North Carolina Department of Health and Human Services at http://www.ncdhhs.gov (accessed 5/31/15).
3. For a description of Osler's work at Hopkins and his creation of the contemporary teaching service, see Michael Bliss, *William Osler: A Life in Medicine* (New York: Oxford University Press, 1999).
4. Rufus Cole, "The Practice of Medicine," *Science* 88, no. 2284 (1938): 312.
5. Cole, "Practice of Medicine," 314.
6. Natalie S. Robins, *The Girl Who Died Twice: Every Patient's Nightmare; The Libby Zion Case and the Hidden Hazards of Hospitals* (New York: Delacorte, 1995), 111.
7. Institute of Medicine (U.S.), Committee on Optimizing Graduate Medical Trainee (Resident) Hours and Work Schedules to Improve Patient Safety, Cheryl Ulmer, Dianne Miller Wolman, and Michael M. E. Johns, *Resident Duty Hours: Enhancing Sleep, Supervision, and Safety* (Washington, D.C.: National Academies Press, 2009).

8. Thomas J. Nasca, Susan H. Day, E. Stephen Amis, and ACGME Duty Hour Task Force, "The New Recommendations on Duty Hours from the ACGME Task Force," *New England Journal of Medicine*, 363, no. 2 (2010): e3.

9. Cole, "Practice of Medicine," 313.

10. See, for example, Christopher P. Landrigan, Amy M. Fahrenkopf, Daniel Lewin, Paul J. Sharek, et al., "Effects of the Accreditation Council for Graduate Medical Education Duty Hour Limits on Sleep, Work Hours, and Safety," *Pediatrics* 122, no. 2 (2008): 250–58; Andrea S. Cedfeldt, Clea English, Raphael El Youssef, Joseph Gilhooly, and Donald E. Girard, "Institute of Medicine Committee Report on Resident Duty Hours: A View from a Trench," *Journal of Graduate Medical Education* 1, no. 2 (2009): 178–80; Teryl K. Nuckols and José J. Escarce, "Cost Implications of ACGME's 2011 Changes to Resident Duty Hours and the Training Environment," *Journal of General Internal Medicine* 27, no. 2 (2012): 241–49; Megha Garg, Brian C. Drolet, Dominick Tammaro, and Staci A. Fischer, "Resident Duty Hours: A Survey of Internal Medicine Program Directors," *Journal of General Internal Medicine* 29, no. 10 (2014): 1349–54; Kiersten Norby, Farhan Siddiq, Malik M. Adil, and Stephen J. Haines, "The Effect of Duty Hour Regulations on Outcomes of Neurological Surgery in Training Hospitals in the United States: Duty Hour Regulations and Patient Outcomes" *Journal of Neurosurgery* 121, no. 2 (2014): 247–61.

Chapter 6. Efficient and Effective

1. Evidence-Based Medicine Working Group, "Evidence-Based Medicine: A New Approach to Teaching the Practice of Medicine," *JAMA* 268, no. 17 (1992): 2424. Guyatt first introduced the phrase a year earlier in Gordon H. Guyatt, "Evidence-Based Medicine," *ACP Journal Club* 114, suppl. 2 (1991): A-16. Sackett and colleagues published a seminal overview for the British medical establishment: David L. Sackett, William M. C. Rosenberg, J. A. Muir Gray, R. Brian Haynes, and W. Scott Richardson, "Evidence-Based Medicine: What It Is and What It Isn't," *BMJ* 312, no. 7023 (1996): 71–72.

2. See Ariel L. Zimerman, "Evidence-Based Medicine: A Short History of a Modern Medical Movement," *Virtual Mentor* 15, no. 1 (2013): 71–76. An insightful oral history of the evidence-based medicine movement was recently published: Richard Smith and Drummond Rennie, "Evidence-Based Medicine—An Oral History," *JAMA* 311, no. 4 (2014): 365–67.

3. Peter C. Wyer and Suzana A. Silva, "Where Is the Wisdom? I—A Conceptual History of Evidence-Based Medicine," *Journal of Evaluation in Clinical Practice* 15, no. 6 (2009): 892.

4. Theodore M. Porter, *Trust in Numbers: The Pursuit of Objectivity in Science and Public Life*. (Princeton, N.J.: Princeton University Press, 1995). Porter provides an overview of his argument in the preface; his statement that "quantification is a technology of distance" can be found on page ix. Further reflections on quantification in medicine can be found in the essay collection edited by Gerard Jorland, Annick Opinel, and George Weisz, *Body Counts: Medical Quantification in Historical and Sociological Perspectives* (Montreal: McGill-Queen's University Press, 2005). The final essays, by George Weisz ("From Clinical Counting to Evidence-Based Medicine") and Theodore Porter ("Medical Quantification: Science, Regulation, and the State"), particularly informed this chapter.

5. Iain Chalmers, "Archie Cochrane (1909–1988)," *Journal of the Royal Society of Medicine* 101, no. 1 (2008): 41–44, available at http://www.ncbi.nlm.nih.gov/pmc/articles/PMC2235918/.

6. Archibald L. Cochrane, *Effectiveness and Efficiency: Random Reflections on Health Services* (London: Nuffield Provincial Hospitals Trust, 1972), 5.

7. Quoted in Clive Adams and Karla Soares, "The Cochrane Collaboration and the Process of Systematic Reviewing," *Advances in Psychiatric Treatment* 3 (1997): 240.

8. Murray Enkin, Marc J. N. C. Keirse, Iain Chalmers, and Eleanor Enkin, *A Guide to Effective Care in Pregnancy and Childbirth*, Oxford Medical Publications (Oxford: Oxford University Press, 1989).

9. The Cochrane organization offers a list of qualifying low- and middle-income countries; see http://community.cochrane.org/editorial-and-publishing-policy-resource/overview-access-options-cochrane-library. For more on the reviews, see Mark Starr, Iain Chalmers, Mike Clarke, and Andrew D. Oxman, "The Origins, Evolution, and Future of the Cochrane Database of Systematic Reviews," *International Journal of Technological Assessment in Health Care* 25, suppl. 1 (2009): 182–95; Joanne E. McKenzie, Georgia Salanti, Steff C. Lewis, and Douglas G. Altman, "Meta-Analysis and the Cochrane Collaboration: Twenty Years of the Cochrane Statistical Methods Group," *Systematic Reviews* 2 (2013): 80.

Chapter 7. Checklists and Dance Lessons

1. See Asaf Degani and Earl L. Wiener, *Human Factors of Flight-Deck Checklists: The Normal Checklist*, ed. Ames Research Center (Moffett Field, Calif.: National Aeronautics and Space Administration, 1990).

2. A cardiac catherization checklist can be found in Srihari S. Naidu, Sunil V. Rao, James Blankenship, Jeffrey J. Cavendish, et al., Society for Cardiovascular Angiography and Interventions, "Clinical Expert Consensus Statement on Best Practices in the Cardiac Catheterization Laboratory: Society for Cardiovascular Angiography and Interventions," *Catheter Cardiovascular Interventions* 80, no. 3 (2012): 456–64.

3. Alex B. Haynes, Thomas G. Weiser, William R. Berry, Stuart R. Lipsitz, et al., and Safe Surgery Saves Lives Study Group, "A Surgical Safety Checklist to Reduce Morbidity and Mortality in a Global Population," *New England Journal of Medicine* 360, no. 5 (2009): 491–99; see also Atul Gawande, *The Checklist Manifesto: How to Get Things Right* (New York: Picador, 2010).

4. See István Ujváry, "Psychoactive Natural Products: Overview of Recent Developments," *Annali dell'Istituto Superiore di Sanità* 50, no. 1 (2014): 12–27.

5. The quality improvement and patient safety literature in medicine is vast, but two of its most important statements are the consensus reports released by the Institute of Medicine: Linda T. Kohn, Janet Corrigan, and Molla S. Donaldson, *To Err Is Human: Building a Safer Health System* (Washington, D.C.: National Academy Press, 2000); and Institute of Medicine (U.S.), Committee on Quality of Health Care in America, *Crossing the Quality Chasm: A New Health System for the Twenty-first Century* (Washington, D.C.: National Academy Press, 2001). A popular account of the quality and safety movement can be found in Charles Kenney, *The Best Practice: How the New Quality Movement Is Transforming Medicine* (New York: Public Affairs, 2008).

6. Lucian L. Leape, "Error in Medicine," *JAMA* 272, no. 23 (1994): 1851–57.

7. See, for example, Mark R. Chassin, Jerod M. Loeb, Stephen P. Schmaltz, and Robert M. Wachter, "Accountability Measures—Using Measurement to Promote Quality Improvement," *New England Journal of Medicine* 363, no. 7 (2010): 683–88.

8. Accreditation Council for Graduate Medical Education, *Common Program Requirements*, 2013. Available at https://www.acgme.org/

acgmeweb/Portals/o/PFAssets/ProgramRequirements/CPRs2013 .pdf (accessed July 31, 2015).

9. John T. James, "A New, Evidence-Based Estimate of Patient Harms Associated with Hospital Care," *Journal of Patient Safety* 9, no. 3 (2013): 122–28.

10. Mark R. Chassin, "Improving the Quality of Health Care: What's Taking So Long?" *Health Affairs (Millwood)* 32, no. 10 (2013): 1762.

11. Deming published several books, but the most relevant are W. Edwards Deming, *Quality, Productivity, and Competitive Position* (Cambridge: Massachusetts Institute of Technology, Center for Advanced Engineering Study, 1982), and *Out of the Crisis* (Cambridge: Massachusetts Institute of Technology, Center for Advanced Engineering Study, 1986).

12. See Hélio A. G. Teive, Guilherme Ghizoni Silva, and Renato P. Munhoz, "Wittgenstein, Medicine and Neuropsychiatry," *Arquivos Neuro-Psiquiatria* 69, no. 4 (2011): 714–16.

13. Charles Taylor, *Philosophical Arguments* (Cambridge: Harvard University Press, 1995).

14. Taylor, *Philosophical Arguments*, 172.

15. See, for example, the essays edited by Renato D. Alarcón, Julia Frank, and Jerome D. Frank, *The Psychotherapy of Hope: The Legacy of Persuasion and Healing* (Baltimore: Johns Hopkins University Press, 2012).

16. Dean Smith, Gerald D. Bell, and John Kilgo, *The Carolina Way: Leadership Lessons from a Life in Coaching* (New York: Penguin, 2004).

Chapter 8. Famous Factory Meatloaf

1. Atul Gawande, "Big Med," *New Yorker*, August 13, 2012, 53. For an example of how members of the quality-improvement movement compare medicine unfavorably to other industrial sites, see Mark R. Chassin and Jerod M. Loeb, "High-Reliability Health Care: Getting There from Here," *Milbank Quarterly* 91, no. 3 (2013): 459–90.

2. Kenneth James, *Escoffier: The King of Chefs* (London: Hambledon and London, 2002).

3. Gawande, "Big Med," 56.

4. Gawande, "Big Med," 54, 60.

5. Gawande, "Big Med," 53.

6. Ivan Illich, *Medical Nemesis: The Expropriation of Health* (New York: Pantheon, 1976).

7. Ivan Illich and David Cayley, *The Rivers North of the Future: The Testament of Ivan Illich* (Toronto: House of Anansi Press, 2005), 204.

8. For examples, see the writings of Donald W. Berwick, a leading figure in the quality and safety movement who recently served as administrator of the Centers for Medicare and Medicaid Services. His influential works include "Continuous Improvement as an Ideal in Health Care," *New England Journal of Medicine* 320, no. 1 (1989): 53–56; Troyen A. Brennan and Donald M. Berwick, *New Rules: Regulation, Markets, and the Quality of American Health Care* (San Francisco: Jossey-Bass, 1996); and Donald M. Berwick, *Promising Care: How We Can Rescue Health Care by Improving It* (San Francisco: Jossey-Bass, 2014).

9. This reading of Foucault is consistent with the interpretations of his work advanced by McKenny and Bishop. See Gerald P. McKenny, *To Relieve the Human Condition: Bioethics, Technology, and the Body* (Albany: State University of New York Press, 1997); Jeffrey Paul Bishop, *The Anticipatory Corpse: Medicine, Power, and the Care of the Dying*, Notre Dame Studies in Medical Ethics (Notre Dame, Ind.: University of Notre Dame Press, 2011).

Chapter 9. Sickbeds and Garden Beds

1. Victoria Sweet, *Rooted in the Earth, Rooted in the Sky: Hildegard of Bingen and Premodern Medicine*, Studies in Medieval History and Culture (New York: Routledge, 2006).

2. Victoria Sweet, *God's Hotel: A Doctor, a Hospital, and a Pilgrimage to the Heart of Medicine* (New York: Riverhead, 2012), 29.

3. Sweet, *God's Hotel*, 5.

4. See Daniel C. Javitt and Robert Freedman, "Sensory Processing Dysfunction in the Personal Experience and Neuronal Machinery of Schizophrenia," *American Journal of Psychiatry* 172, no. 1 (2015): 17–31.

5. Wighard Strehlow and Gottfried Hertzka, *Hildegard of Bingen's Medicine* (Santa Fe: Bear, 1998), 6.

6. Max Weber, *From Max Weber: Essays in Sociology*, trans. Hans Heinrich Gerth and C. Wright Mills (New York: Routledge, 2009), 139.

7. Sharon K. Inouye, "Delirium in Older Persons," *New England Journal of Medicine* 354, no. 11 (2006): 1158.

8. Christian Wiman, *My Bright Abyss: Meditation of a Modern Believer* (New York: Farrar, Straus and Giroux, 2013), 90.

9. *Dartmouth Atlas of Health Care: Tools*, at http://www.dartmouthatlas
.org/tools (accessed May 4, 2015).

Chapter 10. Committed

1. Pierre Rousselot, *The Eyes of Faith*, trans. Joseph Donceel (New York: Fordham University Press, 1990).
2. *Aristotle's Nicomachean Ethics*, trans. Robert C. Bartlett and Susan D. Collins (Chicago: University of Chicago Press, 2011), 26.
3. *Aristotle's Nicomachean Ethics*, 316. This discussion of virtue in medicine is informed by Jennifer Radden and John Z. Sadler, *The Virtuous Psychiatrist: Character Ethics in Psychiatric Practice*, International Perspectives in Philosophy and Psychiatry (New York: Oxford University Press, 2010).
4. Charles L. Bosk, *Forgive and Remember: Managing Medical Failure*, 2nd ed. (Chicago: University of Chicago Press, 2003), 177–78.
5. Jeannette Guerrasio, Maureen J. Garrity, and Eva M. Aagaard, "Learner Deficits and Academic Outcomes of Medical Students, Residents, Fellows, and Attending Physicians Referred to a Remediation Program, 2006–2012." *Academic Medicine* 89, no. 2 (2014): 352–58.
6. See Arthur E. Poropat, "A Meta-Analysis of the Five-Factor Model of Personality and Academic Performance," *Psychological Bulletin* 135, no. 2 (2009): 322–38.
7. For a quantitative sense of how this operates on a national level, see Steven Angus, T. Robert Vu, Andrew J. Halvorsen, Meenakshy Aiyer, et al., "What Skills Should New Internal Medicine Interns Have in July? A National Survey of Internal Medicine Residency Program Directors," *Academic Medicine* 89, no. 3 (2014): 432–35.
8. Christine K. Cassel and James A. Guest, "Choosing Wisely: Helping Physicians and Patients Make Smart Decisions About Their Care," *JAMA* no. 307, no. 17 (2012): 1801–2.
9. Nancy E. Morden, Carrie H. Colla, Thomas D. Sequist, and Meredith B. Rosenthal, "Choosing Wisely—The Politics and Economics of Labeling Low-Value Services," *New England Journal of Medicine* 370, no. 7 (2014): 589–92.
10. Timothy P. Daaleman, Warren A. Kinghorn, Warren P. Newton, and Keith G. Meador, "Rethinking Professionalism in Medical Education Through Formation," *Family Medicine* 43, no. 5 (2011): 326.

Chapter 11. Impatient Attending

1. In Colorado 93 percent of all medical marijuana registrants are registered for "severe pain." See Colorado Department of Public Health and Environment, "Medical Marijuana Registry Program Update, May 31, 2015," at https://www.colorado.gov/pacific/sites/default/files/05_2015_MMR_report.pdf (accessed July 16, 2015).

2. Jerome D. Frank and Julia Frank, *Persuasion and Healing: A Comparative Study of Psychotherapy*, 3rd ed. (Baltimore: Johns Hopkins University Press, 1991). I cite here the third edition, which Jerome Frank co-wrote with his daughter Julia.

3. Frank and Frank, *Persuasion and Healing*, 52.

4. See Scott L. Furney, Alex N. Orsini, Kym E. Orsetti, David T. Stern, et al., "Teaching the One-Minute Preceptor: A Randomized Controlled Trial," *Journal of General Internal Medicine* 16, no. 9 (2001): 620–24. Some of the many teaching tools popular in academic medicine are described in Jennifer R. Kogan, Eric S. Holmboe, and Karen E. Hauer, "Tools for Direct Observation and Assessment of Clinical Skills of Medical Trainees: A Systematic Review," *JAMA* 302, no. 12 (2009): 1316–26.

5. Renato D. Alarcón, Julia Frank, and Jerome D. Frank, eds., *The Psychotherapy of Hope: The Legacy of "Persuasion and Healing"* (Baltimore: Johns Hopkins University Press, 2012).

6. See Tait D. Shanafelt, Sonja Boone, Litjen Tan, Lotte N. Dyrbye, et al., "Burnout and Satisfaction with Work-Life Balance Among US Physicians Relative to the General US Population," *Archives of Internal Medicine* 172, no. 18 (2012): 1377–85.

7. Katherine J. Gold, Ananda Sen, and Thomas L. Schwenk, "Details on Suicide Among US Physicians: Data from the National Violent Death Reporting System," *General Hospital Psychiatry* 35, no. 1 (2013): 45–49.

Chapter 12. Muscle Ups

1. Glassman's analogy can found, among other places, in Andréa Maria Cecil, "Prevention or Prescription?" *CrossFit Journal*, April 6, 2014, available at http://journal.crossfit.com/2014/04/prevention-or-prescription.tpl. The best overview of CrossFit's development is by J. C. Herz, *Learning to Breathe Fire: The Rise of CrossFit and the Primal Future of Fitness* (New York: Crown Archetype, 2014).

2. See, e.g., Stephen J. Bartels, Sarah I. Pratt, Kelly A. Aschbrenner, Laura K. Barre, et al., "Pragmatic Replication Trial of Health Promotion Coaching for Obesity in Serious Mental Illness and Maintenance of Outcomes," *American Journal of Psychiatry* 172, no. 4 (2015): 344–52.

3. For an overview, see Jeanette M. Olsen and Bonnie J. Nesbitt, "Health Coaching to Improve Healthy Lifestyle Behaviors: An Integrative Review," *American Journal of Health Promotion* 25, no. 1 (2010): e1–e12; Ruth Q. Wolever, Leigh Ann Simmons, Gary A. Sforzo, Diana Dill, et al., "A Systematic Review of the Literature on Health and Wellness Coaching: Defining a Key Behavioral Intervention in Healthcare," *Global Advances in Health and Medicine* 2, no. 4 (2013): 38–57; Amireh Ghorob and Thomas Bodenheimer, "Sharing the Care to Improve Access to Primary Care," *New England Journal of Medicine* 366, no. 21 (2012): 1955–57.

4. For example, see Paul Taro Hak, Emil Hodzovic, and Ben Hickey, "The Nature and Prevalence of Injury During CrossFit Training," *Journal of Strength and Conditioning Research* November 22, 2013 (epub ahead of print).

Chapter 13. Doctors Without Silver

1. *Dominican Prayer: Assembly Edition* (Chicago: Dominican Province of St. Albert the Great, 1994), 393.

2. The pamphlets are lost to me now, but the ongoing engagement with Cosmas and Damian was discussed by Jacalyn Duffin in *Medical Saints: Cosmas and Damian in a Postmodern World* (New York: Oxford University Press, 2013); she notes that in 1915 Osler sent a color lithograph of the two saints to the founder of the Mayo Clinic.

3. Stanley Hauerwas, *Suffering Presence: Theological Reflections on Medicine, the Mentally Handicapped, and the Church* (Notre Dame, Ind.: University of Notre Dame Press, 1986), 81.

4. Hauerwas, *Suffering Presence*, 49.

5. David Hilfiker, *Healing the Wounds: A Physician Looks at His Work* (Omaha: Creighton University Press, 1998).

6. For an influential account of the distinction between Platonic and Hippocratic medicine, see Henry Cohen, "The Nature, Methods, and Purpose of Diagnosis," *Lancet* 24, no. 6277 (1943): 23–25.

7. Guenter B. Risse, *Mending Bodies, Saving Souls: A History of Hospitals* (New York: Oxford University Press, 1999), 44.

8. The passage is Micah 6:6–8, from Donald Senior and John J. Collins, eds., *The Catholic Study Bible: The New American Bible, Including the Revised New Testament and Psalms, Translated from the Original Languages with Critical Use of All the Ancient Sources*, 2nd ed. (Oxford: Oxford University Press, 2006), 1287.

9. The passage is Matthew 25:35–36, from Senior and Collins, *Catholic Study Bible*, 1389.

10. The development of Basil's hospital is addressed by Risse, but more fully in Andrew T. Crislip, *From Monastery to Hospital: Christian Monasticism and the Transformation of Health Care in Late Antiquity* (Ann Arbor: University of Michigan Press, 2005).

11. Quoted in Margaret Guenther, *At Home in the World: A Rule of Life for the Rest of Us* (New York: Seabury, 2006), 149.

12. Timothy S. Miller, *The Birth of the Hospital in the Byzantine Empire*, 2nd ed. (Baltimore: Johns Hopkins University Press, 1997).

13. Risse, *Mending Bodies*, 80.

14. Victoria Sweet, *God's Hotel: A Doctor, a Hospital, and a Pilgrimage to the Heart of Medicine* (New York: Riverhead, 2012), 29.

Chapter 14. Red Cards

1. See Martha N. Gardner and Allan M. Brandt, "'The Doctors' Choice Is America's Choice': The Physician in US Cigarette Advertisements, 1930–1953," *American Journal of Public Health* 96, no. 2 (2006): 222–32.

2. Kristen Wyatt, "Colorado Pulls in $76M in Marijuana Taxes and Business Fees for 2014," *Denver Post*, March 10, 2015, available at www.thecannabist.co/2015/02/10/colorado-pot-tax-44-million-recreational-taxes-2014/29510/.

3. Abraham M. Nussbaum, Christian Thurstone, Laurel McGarry, Brendan Walker, and Allison L. Sabel, "Use and Diversion of Medical Marijuana Among Adults Admitted to Inpatient Psychiatry," *American Journal of Drug and Alcohol Abuse* 41, no. 2 (2015): 166–72.

4. The most thorough account of the limited evidence for the medical use of marijuana is Penny F. Whiting, Robert F. Wolff, Sohan Deshpande, Marcello Di Nisio, et al., "Cannabinoids for Medical Use: A Systematic Review and Meta-Analysis," *JAMA* 313, no. 24 (2015): 2456–73. For an overview of the adverse effects of marijuana use, see Nora D. Volkow, Ruben D. Baler, Wilson M. Compton, and Susan R. B. Weiss, "Adverse Health Effects of Marijuana Use," *New England Journal of Medicine* 370, no. 23 (2014): 2219–27.

5. These data come from the Colorado Department of Public Health and Environment and can be accessed online at https://www.colorado.gov/pacific/cdphe/statistics-and-data (accessed August 4, 2015).

6. Talcott Parsons, *The Social System* (London: Routledge, 1991).

7. Nancy Tomes, *Remaking the American Patient: How Madison Avenue and Modern Medicine Turned Patients into Consumers* (Chapel Hill: University of North Carolina Press, 2016). When I was writing this book, I used material from Tomes's book, at that time forthcoming and due for publication in January 2016.

8. For spirited overviews of the rise of our contemporary use of medications, from which these statistics are drawn, see Melody Petersen, *Our Daily Meds: How the Pharmaceutical Companies Transformed Themselves into Slick Marketing Machines and Hooked the Nation on Prescription Drugs* (New York: Farrar, Straus and Giroux, 2008); and David Healy, *Pharmageddon* (Berkeley: University of California Press, 2012).

9. Stanley Hauerwas and Charles Pinches, "Practicing Patience: How Christians Should Be Sick," in *The Hauerwas Reader*, ed. John Berkman and Michael G. Cartwright (Durham, N.C.: Duke University Press, 2001), 348.

10. Annemarie Mol, *The Logic of Care: Health and the Problem of Patient Choice* (London: Routledge, 2008).

11. Christine White and Javier Gonzalez Del Rey, "Decreasing Adverse Events Through Night Talks: An Interdisciplinary, Hospital-Based Quality Improvement Project," *Permanente Journal* 13, no. 4 (2009): 16–22.

Chapter 15. Witnesses

1. There are scores of health inequality papers and textbooks. For a brief illustration of how inequality affects health across generations, see Caroline Sayer and Thomas H. Lee, "Time After Time—Health Policy Implications of a Three-Generation Case Study," *New England Journal of Medicine* 371, no. 14 (2014): 1273–76.

2. See Julie M. Zito, Daniel J. Safer, Devadatta Sai, James F. Gardner, et al., "Psychotropic Medication Patterns Among Youth in Foster Care," *Pediatrics* 121, no. 1 (2008): e157–63.

3. The seven items, known as the "Hospital-Based Inpatient Psychiatric Services Core Measure Set," are created and enforced by the Joint Commission. The list can be accessed at http://www.jointcommission.org/assets/1/6/HBIPS.pdf (accessed July 17, 2015).

4. For example, see Paula W. Yoon, Bastian Brigham, Robert N. Anderson, Janet L. Collins, Harold W. Jaffe, Centers for Disease Control and Prevention, "Potentially Preventable Deaths from the Five Leading Causes of Death—United States, 2008–2010," *MMWR Morbidity and Mortality Weekly Report* 63, no. 17 (2014): 369–74.

5. This literature is reviewed in the summary report by the Institute of Medicine's Committee on Geographic Variation in Health Care Spending and Promotion of High-Value Care, *Variation in Health Care Spending: Target Decision Making, Not Geography,* ed. Joseph P. Newhouse, Alan M. Garber, Robin P. Graham, Margaret A. McCoy, Michelle Mancher, and Ashna Kibria (Washington D.C.: National Academy of Sciences, 2013).

6. Paul Farmer, *Pathologies of Power: Health, Human Rights, and the New War on the Poor* (Berkeley: University of California Press, 2003), 138.

7. Farmer, *Pathologies of Power,* 140.

8. Farmer, *Pathologies of Power,* 157–58.

9. Mission statement, Partners in Health, at http://www.pih.org/pages/our-mission.

10. Farmer, *Pathologies of Power,* 227; Michael Griffin and Jennie Weiss Block, *In the Company of the Poor: Conversations Between Dr. Paul Farmer and Fr. Gustavo Gutiérrez* (Maryknoll, N.Y.: Orbis Books, 2013), 16. The story of Paul Farmer and Partners in Health is also told by Tracy Kidder in *Mountains Beyond Mountains: The Quest of Dr. Paul Farmer, a Man Who Would Cure the World* (New York: Random House, 2003).

11. Paul Farmer and Jonathan Weigel, *To Repair the World: Paul Farmer Speaks to the Next Generation* (Berkeley: University of California Press, 2013), 234.

12. See Alexandra Cook, Joseph Spinazzola, Julian Ford, Cheryl Lanktree, et al., "Complex Trauma in Children and Adolescents," *Psychiatric Annals* 35, no. 5 (2005): 390–98.

13. Jeffrey J. Haugaard, "Recognizing and Treating Uncommon Behavioral and Emotional Disorders in Children and Adolescents Who Have Been Severely Maltreated: Somatization and Other Somatoform Disorders." *Child Maltreatment* 2004, 9(2): 169–76.

14. This history was recently reviewed in Emmanuel Broussolle, Florent Gobert, Teodor Danaila, Stéphane Thobois, Olivier Walusinski, and Julien Bogousslavsky, "History of Physical and 'Moral' Treatment of Hysteria," *Frontiers of Neurology and Neuroscience* 35 (2014): 181–97. The quotation comes from Henry Maudsley, *The Pathology of Mind:*

A Study of Its Distempers, Deformities, and Disorders. (New York: Macmillan, 1895), 138.

Chapter 16. Hope

1. Eric R. Kandel, "A New Intellectual Framework for Psychiatry," *American Journal of Psychiatry* 155, no. 4 (1998): 466.
2. Walker Percy, *Love in the Ruins: The Adventures of a Bad Catholic at a Time Near the End of the World* (New York: Farrar, Straus and Giroux, 1971).
3. Josef Breuer and Sigmund Freud, *Studies on Hysteria* (New York: Basic, 1957), 305.
4. My favorite account of such an approach is the wise book by Margaret Mohrmann, *Medicine as Ministry: Reflections on Suffering, Ethics, and Hope* (Cleveland: Pilgrim, 1995).
5. Sigmund Freud, "Recommendations to Physicians Practicing Psycho-Analysis," in *The Standard Edition of the Complete Psychological Works of Sigmund Freud*, vol.12, ed. James Strachey (London: Hogarth, 1961), 115.
6. Basil of Caesarea, *Ascetical Works*, trans. Sister M. Monica Wagner (New York: Fathers of the Church, 1950), 333.
7. Basil, *Ascetical Works*, 336.

Epilogue

1. Paul R. McHugh, "Striving for Coherence: Psychiatry's Efforts over Classification," *JAMA* 293, no. 20 (2005): 2526–28.
2. P. Eugen Bleuler, "Die Prognose der Dementia praecox (Schizophreniegruppe)," *Allgemeine Zeitschrift für Psychiatrie und psychischgerichtliche Medizin* 65 (1908): 436–64.
3. Walker Percy, *The Moviegoer* (New York: Knopf, 1961), 233. Woods Nash recently reminded me of this passage when he quoted it in his essay, "Searching for Medicine in Walker Percy's *The Moviegoer*," *Literature and Medicine* 31, no. 1 (2013): 114–41.

CREDITS

Portions of Chapters 2 and 10 are reprinted from Abraham M. Nussbaum, "The Faith of a Doctor: Learning to See Beyond the Symptoms," *Commonweal* 134 (2007): 10–14.

Portions of Chapter 4 are reprinted from Abraham M. Nussbaum, "'I Am the Author and Must Take Full Responsibility': Abraham Verghese, the Physicians as the Storytellers of the Body, and the Renewal of Medicine," *Journal of Medical Humanities*, 2014, with kind permission of Springer Science+Business Media.

An earlier version of Chapter 8 was presented at the 2013 Wake Forest Junior Scholars in Bioethics Workshop.

Portions of Chapter 9 are from Abraham M. Nussbaum, "When the Doctor Is a Gardener: Victoria Sweet, Hildegard of Bingen, and the Genres of Physician Writers." Copyright © 2014, The Johns Hopkins University Press. The article first appeared in *Literature and Medicine* 32, no. 2 (Fall 2014): 325–47.

Portions of Chapters 11 and 14 are from A. M. Nussbaum, C. Thurstone, and I. A. Binswanger, "Medical Marijuana Use and Suicide Attempt in a Patient with Major Depressive Disorder," *American Journal of Psychiatry* 168, no. 8 (2011): 778–81, reprinted with permission from *American Journal of Psychiatry* (Copyright © 2011), American Psychiatric Association. All Rights Reserved; and from A. M. Nussbaum, *The Pocket Guide to the DSM-5 Diagnostic Exam* (Arlington, Va.: American Psychiatric Publishing, 2013), reprinted with permission from *The Pocket Guide to the DSM-5 Diagnostic Exam* (Copyright © 2013), American Psychiatric Association. All Rights Reserved.

Portions of Chapter 15 are reprinted from Abraham M. Nussbaum, "The Mennonite Mental Health Movement: Discipleship, Nonresistance, and the Communal Care of People with Mental Illness in Late

Twentieth-Century America" *Journal of Nervous and Mental Disease* 200, no. 12 (2012): 1088–95.

Portions of Chapter 16 are reprinted from Abraham M. Nussbaum, "Changing the Name of Dementia During Residency Training: From Medication Management to CBT to Psychodynamic Psychotherapy," *The Bulletin of the Menninger Clinic* (2011) with permission of The Guilford Press.

INDEX

ABIM Foundation, 160–61
Accreditation Counsel for
  Graduate Medical Education
  (ACGME), 79–80
advertising, 90, 95–96, 216–17
Aequanimitas (Osler), 47, 50
AIDS, 52–54, 61–63
alcohol. *See* intoxication
Allman, Neil, 178–84, 185, 190.
  See also CrossFit
alternative medicine, 138. *See also*
  herbal remedies
American Medical Associa-
  tion (AMA), 75–76, 159–60,
  216–17
AmeriCorps, 192. *See also* Interfaith House
anatomy, 32–36, 50
antipsychotic medications. *See*
  psychiatry: medications used in
appendix, 149
arete, 154. *See also* ethics: virtue
  ethics
Aristotle, 154, 216
"Army Surgeon" (Osler), 48, 50
Arnold P. Gold Foundation,
  42–43
Asclepius, 201
Augustine (saint), 202
authority: for patients' lives
  outside their illness, 255; physi-

cians' decision-making, 7, 8, 63,
  123–24, 214–15
autopsies, 21–23, 26–30, 37. *See
  also* dissection of cadavers

Basil of Caesarea (saint), 203–5,
  237, 254–55
Beaumont, William, 19–21, 22,
  26, 47
Bichat, Marie-François-Xavier, 36
"Big Med" (Gawande), 115, 118,
  124
billing codes, 2, 169. *See also*
  financial aspects of medicine
biological psychiatry, 246. *See also*
  brain; psychiatry
bipolar disorder, 10–11. *See also*
  case histories: Martha
Birth of the Clinic (Foucault), 36
*Birth of the Hospital in the Byzan-
  tine Empire* (Miller), 205
Bishop, Jeffrey, 61–63
bladder/kidney infection, 141
body: encouraging self-healing of,
  134–35, 139–40; as machine,
  1, 30–35, 111, 141 (*see also*
  parts, patients as); meaning of,
  128–29; mortality of, 62, 220,
  221; reading/telling the story
  of, 52–54, 60, 65, 253, 260. *See
  also* patients

physicians (*continued*)
182–83, 254, 260; as technicians, 54, 123–27, 134–35,
196, 253, 260; training of (*see*
medical training); virtue ethics
and, 155; white coats, 38–45,
50; as witnesses, 235, 237–38,
252, 254, 260; workload, 2,
14, 79–82. *See also* diagnosis;
physical examination; physician-
patient relationship
Platonic medicine, 200
poor, the: burdens of illness
suffered disproportionally,
228–29; healthcare services
for, 133, 143, 198–200, 204–6,
227–31 (*see also* Denver Health;
Laguna Honda); reluctance
to care for, 133, 143, 227–28;
tradition of charity/service to,
198–205, 229–31
Porter, Theodore, 88–89
prescription drugs. *See* medications; physicians: as prescribers;
specific medications
primary care physicians, 2–6
professionalism: deficits in,
156–58; and ethics, 215; humanism and, 42–44, 48, 50–51,
63–64; importance of, 67–68;
and the logic of care, 220–21;
and patient choice, 220;
professional distance, 38, 40;
regulation of duty hours and,
80–82; and service, 219 (*see also*
servants, physicians as); white
coat as symbol of, 38–45, 50
psychiatry: algebra analogy, 239,
241, 245; author's decision to

enter, 70–71; author's internship and residency in, 71–75,
84–86, 90, 99–100, 167–70,
239, 246 (*see also* case histories); availability of treatment,
150; complex trauma, 231–32;
consults, 99; contemporary
medicine compared to, 6–7;
Emergency Department, 259;
five-factor model, 158; hospital
psychiatric units, 131–32,
142, 183; medications used in,
72, 77–78, 95–96, 150, 173,
217–18, 261 (*see also specific
medications*); patient assessment,
73–74, 99–100, 131, 162–66,
239, 263; patient goals, 221–22;
questions of exploitation
relevant, 23; self-efficacy, 174;
somatization, 232–33; stigmatization of psychiatric patients,
264; supervision notebook,
167–68; therapeutic alliances,
111, 142, 143, 174, 233–34;
therapeutic techniques,
169–71, 186–87, 243–47,
253–54 (*see also* cognitive
behavioral therapy; psychotherapy); treatment teams,
233. *See also* case histories;
mental illness; *specific mental
illnesses*
psychoanalysis, 246–47, 253–54.
See also case histories: Eleanor
psychodynamic therapy, 246–47
psychotherapy, 167–70, 174,
186–87, 243–44. *See also*
psychiatry
pull-ups, 180–81